Preface

In the 1980s general practitioners worked hard, not only seeing legions of patients but working out-of-hours too (even when they used deputizing services), while records had to be summarized and sorted, appointment systems introduced, staff hired, and nurses and counsellors inducted into the mysteries of family medicine. For those of us working in the inner cities who were trying to catch up with our colleagues in the shire counties, with their group practices and pur pose-built clinics, it was a tough decade. All that changed in the 1990s, when it became obvious that hauling general practice up by its boot-straps was no longer going to be the primary mechanism for developing family medicine. Change came from outside, funding changed from being a means to an end into an end in itself, and the centre of gravity of general practice shifted away from its Royal College towards those who negotiated its contracts. The decade was tough, but in a different way. The election of the New Labour govern ment in 1997 changed the discipline of general practice once again, replacing the crude changes introduced in the nineties with more complex, nuanced and far-reaching reforms. This latter phase of reform has been bewildering for many in general practice, with little to explain what has been happening other than a vague sense among some that the health service is being prepared for privatization, and among others that an essentially sound gatekeeper system of family medicine is being undermined for ideological reasons. Neither expla nation seems satisfactory to me, and each begs more questions than it answers, although I can see that privatization could well be an out come of the reforms.

This book is my attempt to understand what has happened to gen eral practice during my working life in an inner city group practice, and I have started from the perception that family medicine is being industrialized into primary care. This book takes the idea of industri alization literally. I found it difficult to piece together all the different changes that have occurred into a single account of how a health service develops and evolves, and no doubt this difficulty shows. Each piece of the jigsaw has been tried in many places, in the hope that it would make a recognizable image and contribute to a coherent picture. Not every piece fits properly, and some readers may suggest alternative images that will coalesce into a different picture. That would be welcome, because this book is exploratory and has taken me into unfamiliar and sometimes uncomfortable subjects. I have tried to understand and apply different sociological perspectives, some ideas from political economy and the insights of a range of other disciplines to explain the trends in general practice that I have experienced, and no doubt I have missed out useful data and theories in doing so. This attempt to understand the recent history of family medicine has not been easy, because Universities encourage their academics to stay inside their silos and—with some exceptions—not to stray across boundaries. Although many academic general practitioners have investigated aspects of recent changes in their discipline, no academic department or organization has tried to develop even a partial overview, with the exception of the National Primary Care Research & Development Centre at the University of Manchester.

This disappointment has been offset by three sources of inspiration. My practice colleagues have, over nearly three decades, debated and argued endlessly about change in general practice. The collective effort to make sense of what was going on around us, being done to us, and being constructed through our work was practical not scholarly, but it fuelled a sense of enquiry and an enduring scepticism about received wisdom, and I am grateful for this. Another small group, the European section of the International Association for Health Policy (IAHPE), provided the environment for discussing the politics of change in health services. I am particularly grateful to Uli Deppe, Alexis Benos, Mauri Johansson, and Finn Diderichsen for their wide knowledge, political wisdom and critical thinking, and am well aware that they will not agree with all of my arguments. The debates in IAHPE led to the publication of early attempts to understand the industrialization of family medicine, first in the Spanish public health bulletin *Quadern Caps* and later in the *Journal of Public Health Policy*, spurring me on to extend the exploration. Finally, some of my academic colleagues have contributed to and sometimes challenged

From General Practice to Primary Care

The industrialization
of family medicine

From General Practice to Primary Care
The industrialization of family medicine

Steve Iliffe

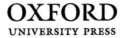

OXFORD
UNIVERSITY PRESS

OXFORD
UNIVERSITY PRESS

Great Clarendon Street, Oxford OX2 6DP

Oxford University Press is a department of the University of Oxford.
It furthers the University's objective of excellence in research, scholarship,
and education by publishing worldwide in

Oxford New York

Auckland Cape Town Dar es Salaam Hong Kong Karachi
Kuala Lumpur Madrid Melbourne Mexico City Nairobi
New Delhi Shanghai Taipei Toronto

With offices in

Argentina Austria Brazil Chile Czech Republic France Greece
Guatemala Hungary Italy Japan Poland Portugal Singapore
South Korea Switzerland Thailand Turkey Ukraine Vietnam

Oxford is a registered trade mark of Oxford University Press
in the UK and in certain other countries

Published in the United States
by Oxford University Press Inc., New York

British Library Cataloguing in Publication Data

Data available

Library of Congress Cataloging-in-Publication Data

Data available

Typeset by Cepha Imaging Private Ltd., Bangalore, India
Printed in Great Britain
on acid-free paper by
Biddless Ltd., King's Lynn, Norfolk

ISBN 978–0–19–921450–1

10 9 8 7 6 5 4 3 2 1

Contents

the thinking behind this book, although not always knowingly. James Munro, the editor of *Health Matters*, asked lots of difficult questions and invariably had another angle on events and their causes. Vari Drennan and Claire Goodman, both knowledgeable in health services research, have been consistently good natured and helpful about my forays into disciplines other than medicine. Jill Manthorpe brought a well-grounded social perspective to every discussion about general practice that I have had with her, and kindly led me away from the murky depths of post-modern sociology, among other traps. Trish Labro sourced material, corrected chapters and produced bound manuscripts over many months, and put up with the unreasonable deadlines I sometimes gave her. None of these people are to blame for this book.

Steve Iliffe FRCGP
Lonsdale Medical Centre, London NW6
and
the Department of Primary Care & Population Sciences,
University College London.
16 July 2007

Introduction

In *Hippocratic oaths*[1] Professor Raymond Tallis writes '... if we are not careful, the patient-as-client will receive service-with-a-smile from a "customer-aware" self-protecting doctor delivering strictly on contract ... medicine may become the first blue-collar profession, delivered by supine, sessional functionaries.' Professor Tallis goes on, in an article in *The Times*,[2] to castigate the corrupting effects of incentives, targets, and managerial interference in clinical care that create 'a parallel world of delivery that is remote from the real world.' Another Professor, gynaecologist James Owen Drife, reports how his wife (a general practitioner) has taken up learning Russian as light relief from the bureaucracy of general practice, and how his experience of being managed makes him (and his fellow practitioners) into sullen serfs who only realize what is happening to them and to the National Health Service (NHS) 'at meetings of the Royal College of Serfs.'[3] Something is happening within medicine to make those at the top of the professional pyramid very distressed indeed.

In general practice this distress seems to be felt even more acutely, perhaps because the ethos of general practice emphasizes the importance of long-term personable relationships between doctor and patient that foster trust, allow open communication and permit the free exchange of ideas and information. Dougal Jeffries, writing in the *British Journal of General Practice*, says: 'From a profession distinguished by its variety of independent practitioners, all bringing their own ideas and approaches to bear on their daily work, we are being turned into a homogeneous regiment of government agents, bribed and browbeaten into toeing the party line.'[4] *Doctor* newspaper, surveying the views of 600 GPs in the autumn of 2006, noted complaints about interference by Primary Care Trusts in clinical practice, the substitution of less trained staff for experienced practitioners, the adverse effects of protocols on the art of medicine, and the subversion of the clinical decision agreement between doctor and patient by accountants.[5]

There are dark forces at work behind this subversion of professionalism. London GP Iona Heath, writing in the *British Medical Journal* in 2007, attributes the separation of day and night primary care services to the government's wish to 'break the GP monopoly and to open up GP services to commercial competition'.[6] Echoing this Ian Quigley, a GP in Romford, argues for a *volte face* in policy, so that the government should 'make GPs work evenings and weekends. And then leave us alone for ten years. Please'.[7] This desire to go back to the old form of general practice fits within a broader feeling about health service policy, neatly summed up by Professor Alyson Pollock: 'Nothing but a complete reversal of policy will save the NHS.'[8] This fear of privatization is a profound one that arises in part from the fundamentally antimarket stance of general practice that I will return to later. The desire to turn the clock back, and to restore the old order, is one I will revisit in the last chapter of this book.

Patients can be similarly afflicted with this anguish. One example of patient distress from among many magazine articles, television programmes and books is Sophie Petit-Zeman's *Doctor, what's wrong? Making the NHS human again.*[9] It confronts the industrialism of:

> ... a medical machine (that is) spinning out of control. As it gets bigger, in some ways better, bringing more people more chance of better lives, are those who work within it, those who care, losing the will and ability to do so? Pushed into robot-mode by managers with books to balance and targets to meet, some feel close to breaking point, while the huge, impersonal system levies the self-seeking free to cheat it, unnoticed, more easily than before. And lost in the melée: patients.

The industrialization of medicine is seen as a malignant phenomenon that negates the individuality of the patient and the creativity of the doctor, turning the former into the object of a production-line process, and making the latter give up a craft in favour of clinical practice driven by protocols, guidelines, and evidence-based medicine.

The industrialization of medicine

The anxieties appear to be widespread, even affecting some users of the health service, and seem to go to the core of professional self-identity. Medicine is changing from a craft concerned with the uniqueness of each encounter with an ill person to a mass-manufacturing industry preoccupied with the throughput of the sick. Doctors (and no doubt other professionals, but we hear little of them) are becoming proletarians, not artisans, changing the colour of their collar from white to blue. The strength of professional feeling is intense, as if doctors were being dispossessed, driven out of their comfortable little workshops into huge factories in an industrial revolution over which they have no control. The fear of professionals is that their work will deteriorate in quality, and that the ill people and the society that they serve will receive a poorer service because of the managerial efforts to reorganize and standardize clinical practice, increase productivity and above all, break even.

This dramatic tale of high-speed industrialization certainly makes good news stories for tabloids and entertaining fillers for learned journals, but it may not be true. At least, not true in the sense described by its apparent victims. Professors Tallis and Drife talk of an emerging Soviet system, not because they have a scholarly knowledge of that system and see the warning signs within the NHS, but because recycling myths about totalitarian control is their way of emphasizing the seriousness and intensity of the changes they are experiencing. Dougal Jeffries joins them in his fear of being made to 'toe the party line'. They are going beyond the idea of industrialization, and hint at obedience, conformity, and even slavery.

This is obviously hyperbole, but why do professionals whose judgements in their clinical work are likely to be informed, cautious, and considered making claims about imminent slavery that are arguably extreme, exaggerated, and ill-informed? One possibility is that they have a political agenda, echoing the accusations of 'Stalinism' that Conservative Party makes against the NHS from time to time, as a way of showing its hostility to Big Government and its yearning for a more commercialized medical environment where choice (and the financial resources needed for it) will shape the service. This may be true for some complainants, but probably not for all; my experience of colleagues who have given up general practice in recent years, blaming one or other aspect of the industrialization of medicine, is that they did not lack commitment to the public health service, but did feel that it lacked commitment to them.

Patrician disdain?

It could also be due to a patrician disdain of the managerial lower orders, an almost aristocratic refusal to be told what to do by lesser, non-clinical, beings, that arises when a particular social order with medicine at its apex is challenged. This may be closer to the truth, reflecting a struggle for power over the control of resources—working time, staffing levels, access to imaging or operating theatres or highly specialized therapies—but then it is nothing new. The balance of power between professionals and the funders of health services has been a see-saw since the days of Bismark, let alone Bevan. Prophecies of the death of civilized medical care are then just part of the profession's counter-attack against overweening State power, and like shroud-waving and other techniques for rallying opinion can be discounted as no more than battle cries that will subside once this particular struggle is decided.

If this were true then the warnings about slavery would be coming from the political class within medicine, and the mass of practitioners would applaud occasionally but without giving the claims too much critical attention, and then get on with their jobs. In this book I will explore this possibility—that we are observing just a particular style of political theatricality—but at the beginning I have little conviction that it is true. It is the widespread discontent, the breadth and depth of feeling, and the entry into the argument of thoughtful and critical thinkers such as Professor Tallis, that make me feel that there is something else happening, and that the industrialization of medicine—and in particular, of general practice—is a real phenomenon.

An illegible reality

The proclaimed Sovietization of the NHS is a symptom of an underlying process but not a sensible description, let alone a diagnosis. Here lies the problem, because—tabloids and fillers aside—there is little detailed, analytic description of the industrialization of medicine in the medical or sociological literature. Descriptions of some of the symptoms—effects of incentives and targets, the impact of reorganization, or the consequences of perverse incentives—are abundant, but the unifying idea of industrialization with its own internal dynamics and logic is largely missing. This does not mean that there is no industrialization process underway in medicine, and that learned Professors and jobbing GPs are merely being swept up in a wave of histrionic reactions to changes in their working environments. Richard Sennett reminds us that the most basic cultural problem of our time is that 'much of modern social reality is illegible to the people trying to make sense of it.'[10]

This book is an attempt to make the illegible legible, using five propositions about the changes that we have experienced. The first is that a qualitative change in the orientation and organization of British general practice began around 1990. Many changes that had begun sometimes long before that date, like the growth of group practices, the development of multidisciplinary teamwork, the introduction of appointment systems and the outsourcing of night and weekend working, were incorporated into the change, but the change was much more than the sum of these parts. This change is what we are experiencing as industrialization.

The second is that while the independent contractor status of British GPs put us at arm's length from the public sector, we remained firmly within what David Marquand describes as the public realm.[11] The changes that began around 1990 contain a great deal of what Marquand calls 'market mimicry', the adoption of market ideas or mechanism, but their combined effect is to draw general practice much closer to the public sector, or even into it. The actual relationship between the changes that we are experiencing and the much-feared privatization is unclear. Are the changes that are now occurring in general practice a form of privatization, a precursor and preparation for future privatization, or only risks for privatization with other outcomes still possible?

The third proposition is that the changes that we have experienced in the last two decades fit with the view that multiple changes in routines, customs, practices, and ways of working can accumulate (sometimes in unexpected ways) and break the framework of rules, funding arrangements and organizational structures that we have taken for granted, often with unpredictable outcomes. The most recent expression of this view of change comes from Roberto Unger, a Brazilian lawyer turned historian and sociologist of change,[12] but has a long pedigree in dialectical thinking about social development. The particular quality that Unger brings to thinking about change is the awareness that outcomes cannot be predetermined with any accuracy, that unintended consequences can weigh more than intended ones, and that social existence is fuzzy and messy, a feeling that seems to me to fit well with our everyday experience of general practice.

The fourth proposition is that the pattern of changes that we are experiencing is recognisably similar to the process that converted engineering as a profession from a craft discipline to an industrial one. This industrialization process is not planned, but emerges as a multitude of small changes, each logical in its own terms, coalesce into a major social shift. These comparisons between engineers' experiences in the late nineteenth and early twentieth centuries with ours in the late twentieth and early twenty-first centuries will, I hope, reveal how industrialization processes are changing person-centred family medicine into system-centred primary care. The main components of this transformation of engineering from a craft activity to an industrial one are:

1. The growth of management.
2. The incorporation of the distribution network for goods into the industry that makes them, a process of 'forward integration'.
3. The adoption of large volume, continuous production methods.
4. The adoption of efficient, production line ways of working, including the subdivision of labour, the standardization of techniques, the replacement of people by machines, and the incentivization and speed-up of work processes.
5. The incorporation of science into the industry through the codification of knowledge and the engagement of scientists in the management of the industry.

GPs (and hospital specialists) may recognize some feature of their current working life in this list. I will try to translate each into the history and vocabulary of general practice in the chapters of this book, to test the idea that we are indeed living through a process of (increasingly rapid) industrialization. For each component of change I will ask whether there are alternatives that might preserve the relationships that are necessary for personalized medical care alongside the science and technology that make it effective.

The fifth proposition is that the way in which general practice is funded and the way in which we relate to the NHS shapes clinical activity and the organization of our practices more than professional commitments to the well-being of patients or the equity of the provision of medical care. This is not to say that, using Julian Le Grand's terms,[13] we are necessarily more like knaves (concerned with our own well-being) than knights (concerned with the welfare of others), but it is to argue that general practice tends towards being institutionally conservative in its thinking about how to develop, despite strong professional counter-currents favouring innovation.

Primary care

General practice in the UK is being industrialized into primary care. The process of change is not a mere reorganization, but a transformation of an activity from a loosely organized enterprise with a poorly defined remit and wide scope for individual initiative, interpretation and innovation, into a predictable and prescribed series of tasks in the management of the public's health. It is creating anxieties among professionals about power, autonomy, and patient-centeredness as well as concern among citizens about the motivations of professionals. It offers the prospect of a standardized service, performing in the same way in Brighton as in Barnsley for the wide range of expectations, understandings and experiences found among the critical, informed (or misinformed), anxious citizens of what Anthony Giddens calls 'high modern society'.[14] And it is widely (if understandably) misunderstood, with its symptoms—targets for immunization of pre-school children, appointments available within 48 hours, for example—attracting more attention than its underlying causes. This book attempts to explain what industrialization means when applied to health services, and in particular to the transformation of British general practice from 'family medicine' to 'primary care'. It is concerned with general practice as a form of work, a productive process that can create a range of end products, from the renewal or maintenance of health to the sustenance of social stability itself.

When seen from an organizational or business standpoint, health services are multi-unit enterprises providing multicomponent services, organizationally equivalent to very large, diversified companies. Although public health services such as Britain's NHS are not for-profit enterprises, they may share some characteristics with commercial companies, particularly where these characteristics offer methods of cost-containment. Cost-containment in health services is not simply an expression of a neo-liberal perspective on healthcare, and will not leave the policy agenda. A health service that is not organized on principles that attempt to extract the biggest gain out of any set of resources is conceivable at the beginning of the twenty-first century, but it seems unlikely to be something that we will experience. Even if there is a major change in public thinking about how the wealth of the nation is spent, so that resources shift from personal and private consumption to public provision, mechanisms will be needed to ensure that this abundance is not exploited by relative outsiders (such as the pharmaceutical industry) or insiders such as professionals seeking more pay for less work. The history of the NHS is a cyclic one of cost-containment mechanisms being weakened and strengthened, from the abolition and reintroduction of charges to patients that prompted Bevan's resignation in 1951, through the cash limits imposed after the oil crisis in the 1970s, to the period of expanded funding from 2003 to 2008 following the restrictions of the 1990s.

As all health services, however organized, face the same problem of resources being insufficient to keep up with growing demand for healthcare. They exhibit an underlying tendency towards solving problems using mechanisms borrowed from other industries, particularly the disciplinary force of market mechanisms. We should note the observation of Raymond Williams that:[15]

> An economy is determined by its major dominant structure and what has hopefully taken out to work on different principles is eventually drawn back into the major orbit, or is at best made marginal and, in its explicit funding, vulnerable. We have seen this, since the sixties, in case after case, where commercial standards and priorities have been steadily re-imposed.

What kind of market?

Commercial development follows its own logic, and governments may have only a limited impact in shaping that logic. The brief respite from neo-liberal policies in healthcare in some parts of Europe at the end of the 1990s (for example with the election of New Labour in the UK, Schroeder's government in Germany and the Olive Coalition in Italy), did not bring about an end to the tendency to solve problems in healthcare using market approaches, methods, and mechanisms, (although many of their supporters thought it should have done so), but it did alter the approaches, methods and mechanisms used. The question became not: Market or not? But instead: What kind of market?

As we shall see in the following chapters, Britain's government since 1997 has grasped how useful particular kinds of market mechanisms could be within a highly managed industry in which a diverse range of professionals supply a spectrum of services to an increasingly differentiated society. We shall see how this change in policy shifted health service management away from the failed model of fundholding and the industrial market tried between 1991 and 1999, towards a managed market in which all components of the NHS 'industry' are tied together by economic links designed to keep a complex network of services viable, but only if they function efficiently. We shall return to the meanings of 'function' and 'efficiently' in subsequent chapters, after reviewing the evolution of general practice as an economic activity in Chapter 1, and seeing how the industrialization process is transforming it. The key concepts in Chapter 1 are the nature of franchises, the strengths and weaknesses of co-operatives, the limits of a trading market (the fundholding experiment), and the reversion to an industrial, managed market under New Labour. I do not apologize for the lengthy discussion of fundholding, because its failure set the scene for the introduction of the new General Medical Services (GMS) contract of 2004, which is accelerating the process of industrialization in general practice.

The pattern of industrialization

The industrialization process is following a traditional pattern, described in detail in Chapters 2–6. Chapter 2 describes how in large, complex industries market and price mechanisms are internalized, taking the form of management. Developing commercial industries replace the purchase of raw materials, labour, expertise, and distribution mechanisms in open markets with increasingly complex management structures that supervise the acquisition, production and distribution of products, and then fix prices. They become national or international corporations, or even monopolies. The preoccupation of the NHS with management reorganization makes sense when understood as an effort to bring market trading under control, and to maximize the value extracted from every pound spent, every hour worked, every encounter between professional and patient. This has profound implications for general practice, which has to come to terms first with the shift from the administration of a franchise to the management of a contract, and then with the progressive redefinition of that contract. Practice-based commissioning is an expression of this process, making GPs part of the purchasing mechanism in the developing industrial market, beneficiaries of its successes but also answerable for its failures.

Forward integration, mass production

Chapter 3 describes the process of 'forward integration' with incorporation of a distribution network into the structure of the industry. Part of the process of internalization of markets includes taking control, where necessary, of suppliers and distributors, to make them more responsive to the needs of the industry. For example, a mobile phone company can rely on generic shops to sell mobile phones, or open its own. For general practice forward integration has meant that we have moved from an arms-length relationship with the NHS to a closer connection, with some practices being run directly by Primary Care Trusts, others bound by specific, locally determined contracts (PMS practices) and a third group tied to the NHS by an elaborate and evolving franchise contract (GMS practices). The contracts have shifted from individuals (who can work collectively as they choose) to groups, and from capitation and fee-based remuneration systems towards payment by results, the Quality and Outcomes Framework being a typical example. The subdivision of labour, with ever-greater specialization, the construction of new disciplines and the re-writing of job roles in existing professional groups, are other expressions of this process.

Chapter 4 outlines how an expanding, increasingly integrated industry adopts large-batch, continuous-process technologies, replacing individualized, craft production by mass production, with an emphasis on the volume of output. In general practice this appears as the standardization of tools, with its emphasis on concordance with guidelines for best practice. The individuality of the patient is not ignored or avoided, but it is subordinated to the systematic application of scientific knowledge. The idiosyncracies of the person with diabetes are not allowed to over-ride the need for their treatment regimen to be optimized, and for their risks of serious, disabling, potentially life-threatening and costly complications to be reduced. One diabetic individual's eating habits are less important than the blood glucose control of all those registered with the practice. The wider use of incentive payments to change activity or increase productivity, exemplified by the new contract for general practice introduced in 2004, is an example of this, as is the pressure to speed up work processes, by setting deadlines and targets for achieving clinically desirable objectives such as smoking cessation, influenza immunization, and so on.

Chapter 5 focuses on the need to maximize efficiency in family medicine, with the application of Taylorist (efficient working practices) and Fordist (production line) approaches in management, the design of work sites, and the organization of work processes. These approaches are characterized by the central codification of knowledge, expressed in the shape of evidence-based medicine, a set of rules about what works and what does not work in medicine and nursing, and the substitution of human skills with machines, best seen in general practice in the ubiquitous desk-top computer and its decision-support software. All of these features of industrialization are now becoming part of everyday general practice, and causing widespread unease among professionals.

Utopian ideology and clinical governance

Chapter 6 demonstrates how science is incorporated into the industry, through linkage of professionals with the corporate interests of the industry itself. A utopian ideology that emphasizes the benefits of the application of science to society, in the form being promoted by the health industry, emerges and becomes powerful. In the NHS this ideology is 'clinical governance', and this chapter will explore the meanings of clinical governance and the consequences of its spread within primary care. Career paths are created for scientists to enter management within the industry, some in clinical governance roles and some through practice-based commissioning—both different ways in which practitioners can pick up and carry risks while also wielding some (limited) local power.

What about the patients? No part of this story so far has included those who use primary care in a decisive, shaping role. Public expectations are cited as reasons to want, or not want changes in general practice, and polling opinion is now built into the new GP contract. How important is this trend to public involvement, and how does it fit alongside the industrialization process? Chapter 7 will review the empirical evidence about medical consumerism and its mirror image, 'producerism' (doctor and patient as co-producer of health) and examine how challenges to medical authority on the one hand and participatory democracy on the other are used to discipline general practice.

My argument is that using this model of industrialization as an analytic framework has two advantages. It explains the sometimes complex development of British general practice over time, in a way that integrates economics, organization, professional ideology and medical science, and suggests coherence in processes of change that can appear mysterious and incoherent. And it explains the failure of the market reforms of 1991–9, which adopted models of development exactly opposite to those of historic industrialization. Instead of forward integration of distributors of medical care (GPs) and Fordist standardization of work processes the market reforms introduced by Conservative governments emphasized the retail function of small-scale producers. Although there was an increase in administration in general practices, it was concerned with comparing prices, shopping round and invoicing, not the internalization of market mechanisms. The current reforms correspond much more closely to the industrialization model described, with incorporation of previously franchised GPs into a more precisely described and tightly managed production process.

Are there alternatives?

Chapter 8 asks if this industrialization process is 'a good thing', and what alternatives (if any) might exist. The transformation of general practice into primary care appears to have huge advantages. The standard of medical care in the community seems likely to rise and the dramatic variations in clinical activity seem likely to decrease as the principles of 'best practice' become core components of contracts. Evidence-based medicine allows fewer and fewer doctors to hide behind idiosyncratic treatments or simple ignorance. Governance rules require more and more clinicians to incorporate the perspective of social responsibility—the common use of the common wealth—into their thinking about disease, illness, and the demands of their case load. Information technology has transformed everyday work and made knowledge from every clinical encounter accessible, understandable, and usable for clinical problem-solving, education, and research. Industrialization's advocates will tell us that we should be pleased to see such changes occurring, and put our energies into promoting them.

However, there problems with industrialization processes in medicine that we need to understand. Such industrial development has not taken place in all large-scale enterprises, even in the USA and certainly not in mainland Europe, partly because it may be resisted by employers and industrial managers alike. It may work only in expanding economies, and it does not necessarily satisfy consumers or service users. Industrial processes in medicine may lead to the objectification of the citizen, and simple linear solutions being applied to complex, systemic problems in an impersonal, deskilled, rule-driven environment. Within family medicine there are fears about loss of professional identity, commitment to whole person medicine, and the advocacy role, and therefore there is resistance to the changes. Even if we disagree with this perspective, we need to take it seriously and think it through. If maximal industrialization occurs in general practice we might see:

1. The growth of a professionally diversified workforce, with increasing part-time working, and a target-driven, impersonal work style with limited responsiveness to individuals and evident rationing of services.

2. Large-scale skill transfers, with nurse practitioners becoming alternatives to doctors and minimally trained staff (healthcare assistants) taking on simple nursing tasks.

3. The growth of the private medical sector, which will claim to offer the personalized service that the public sector is losing. (This is likely to be a spurious claim, as the growth of the private sector is also likely to result in industrialization processes occurring within it).

4. The further growth of 'alternative medicine', which will be genuinely personal as long as it is based on individual practitioners.

However, if the medical profession in Britain is able to resist these trends and a form of responsible autonomy is retained by practitioners, there is likely to be less standardization of primary care services, and apparently inescapable variations in the quality of practice. A slower pace of change in the organization of general practice and in the diffusion of knowledge and expertise will follow, with professional resistance to rationalization of services and cost containment. This will produce continuous conflict between professions and government over resource allocation, and possibly a renewal of interest in patient-centredness as an ideology of practice, best exemplified at present by the current fashion for 'narrative-based medicine'. Compromises between industrialization and craft work that try to tailor the standardized science to individuals are emerging, such as 'personal management plans' and 'goal-oriented medical practice'. Similarly, approaches such as Community Oriented Primary Care seek to engage citizens and professionals in the dialogues necessary to match service provision to the complexities and sheer messiness of the health problems of real communities, but at a social rather than individual patient level.

These alternatives to industrialization do nothing to address the issue of resources and demand, and may be little more than a route to conflict between professionals and politicians, with failure to change the performance and character of public health services. Given the tendency to find compromise solutions at micro-, meso-, and macro-levels within the healthcare system, Unger would predict that such conflicts may appear and be resolved piecemeal (and perhaps only partially) over a long period of time. In a worst case scenario the undoubted benefits of the industrialization of family medicine may not be so apparent against a backdrop of professional discontent and political conflict. If this occurs then privatization of primary care would appear to be a solution, to retain maximal services for those who can afford them and minimal, safety-net services for those who cannot. In a best case scenario piecemeal and partial adaptations of the industrialization process, enriched by goal- and community-oriented approaches, will invigorate general practice with new ways to merge scientific knowledge and the personal relationships at the centre of family medicine. Which way will we go?

References

1. Tallis R. *Hippocratic oaths*. London: Atlantic Books, 2004.
2. Tallis R. Targets have failed the NHS. *The Times* 2006; **10 August.**
3. Drife JO. All Russian to me. *BMJ* 2006; **333**: 865.
4. Jeffries D. Ever been HAD? *Br J Gen Pract* 2006; 392.
5. Ford S. GPs fear demise of profession's status. *Doctor* 2006; **24 October.**
6. Heath I. Out of hours primary care—a shambles? *BMJ* 2007; **334**: 341.
7. Quigley I. How much are doctors really worth: how much do doctors really earn? *BMJ* 2007; **334**: 343.
8. Quoted in: Kmietowicz Z One year to save the NHS: what would you do? *BMJ* 2007; **334**: 181.
9. Petit-Zeman S. *Doctor, what's wrong? Making the NHS human again.* Routledge, 2005.
10. Sennett R. *The culture of the New Capitalism.* Yale University Press, 2006, pp. 11–12.
11. Marquand D. *The decline of the public.* Cambridge: Polity Press, 2005.
12. Unger RM. *False necessity.* London: Verso, 2004.
13. Le Grand J. *Motivation, agency and public policy: of knights and knaves, pawns and queens.* Oxford University Press, 2003.
14. Giddens A. *Modernity and self identity: self and society in the late modern age.* Cambridge: Polity Press, 2002.
15. Williams R. *What I came to say.* London: Hutchinson Radius, 1990, p. 103.

Chapter 1

The political economy of family medicine

Doctors ... are not rationally calculating market actors, behaving in accordance with the profit motive—or, at any rate, not solely. At least in principle they are supposed to abide by an ethic of public service that tells them to pursue the public interest, even if they earn their living in a market of some sort.

David Marquand, Decline of the Public (2004)

It is difficult to know when the processes of industrialization began to have an impact on general practice. Frank Honigsbaum's history of the separation of general practice and specialist medicine in Britain[1] in the first half of the twentieth century describes the culture of competition, conflict, and complaint that dominated medical practice, with general practitioners (GPs) critical of bureaucracy when the local Panel was difficult or demanding, and the strife did not disappear after 1948, with the foundation of the National Health Service (NHS). Now we complain about filling in ever more forms, meeting targets, completing the paperwork needed to fulfil legal obligations as employers and 'governance' obligations as professionals. We are uncomfortable with 'ticking boxes', 'jumping through hoops' and practising 'medicine by numbers', but we may also be unsure exactly when all this discontent began. Was it in 1966 with the Family Doctors' Charter, in 1990 with the contract imposed on GPs by the Department of Health, or only recently with New Labour's modernizing zeal and seemingly unending flurry of reforms?

Our experience is only part of the picture of industrialization. If we take another symptom, the impersonality of medical care, we could see this either as a new arrival, driven by the most recent changes, or as a fundamental feature of the system within which we work. We may describe ourselves as providing personal and continuing care to individuals and families, but our actual behaviour will probably lie along a spectrum from personalized to anonymous, and we may not position ourselves on that spectrum in the place an outside observer would choose. For example, a comparative study of British and French general practice described British GPs as providing delayed, impersonal, and good quality medical care while their French peers (who worked much longer hours with fewer patients) provided immediate, personal, and good quality care.[2] We know about this impersonality, of course, and respond to its negative effects by retraining doctors emerging into general practice from hospital medicine, and by emphasizing the importance in practice and research of consultation styles and techniques. This focus on doctor–patient interactions must be one of the great successes of general practice in Britain, as is the role that GPs have played in creating space within undergraduate curricula for communication skills training.

For the purposes of this book the symptoms of industrialization are less important than the recognition of the syndrome itself, the collection of changes that hint at a process of change that is well underway by the time it is noticed, and that threatens or promises to shape the future. There are a number of reasons to think that the industrialization syndrome appeared at about 1990, and we will return to them throughout the book. For example, Rudolf Klein, an eminent commentator on the health service, argued that the NHS policy announcements of 1989 amounted to 'a turning point in the history of the NHS, a deliberate repudiation of the past …',[3] which GPs experienced directly with the unilateral imposition of a new contract for general practice in 1990. This is where I want to start the story of industrialization. Before I do that, however, I want to explore industrialization's prehistory on the grounds that the organization of general practice, and the expectations and attitudes of GPs, have influenced the ways in which industrialization took hold and transformed general practice into primary care at the end of the twentieth century.

My argument is that developments in British general practice can be seen as occurring in three phases: (1) a long phase of evolution from 1948 to 1990; (2) a short period of attempted market reform, from 1991 to 1999; and (3) a reversion to control and planning after 1999, but with increasing use of market mechanisms to engineer changes in the organization of services. Industrialization as a process emerged in the middle phase, through the 1990s, and followed a turbulent course before stabilizing and becoming entrenched in general practice after 1997, producing an experience (from the inside) of accelerating change. The long-term trends in the organization of British general practice between 1948 and 1990 are shown in Table 1.1.[4,5]

There are two aspects of this period of evolution that are relevant to this book. The first is that industrialization has accelerated some processes, such as the separation of in-hours and out-of-hours work, and reversed others, such as falling list sizes. The pattern of evolution of general practice established in the two decades after the formation of the NHS is changing. The second is that during this period British general practice functioned as a franchise, with all the advantages and disadvantages of this form of industrial organization.

Table 1.1 Long-term trends in British general practice

- Group formation: solo practice becomes uncommon, and almost synonymous with poor clinical performance.
- Appointments systems: direct access to medical care is controlled by administrative staff and appointment systems.
- Falling lists sizes: each doctor has fewer registered patients.
- Increased staffing: each doctor has more support workers, and the range of disciplines working in primary care increases.
- Withdrawal from out-of-hours work (especially in the cities), and maternity care, occur. Both of these parts of clinical work are delegated, the first to a group of doctors who choose to do night and weekend work (or who can find no other employment), and the second to hospital obstetricians and midwives.
- Child health and contraception are 'colonized' as areas of generalist rather than specialist expertise.
- Delegation of chronic disease management to nurses.

Franchise development

There is a tendency, even within otherwise perceptive academic institutions such as the National Primary Care Research & Development Centre at the University of Manchester to think of general practice as an independent business, taking a cue from the profession's own description of itself as an 'independent contractor' to the NHS. Aside from believing too readily the account that any organization gives of its place and role in society, we can see very easily how inaccurate the 'independent business' description is. Since 1948 general practice has been dependent on a monopoly funder, the NHS, with no significant alternative source of income. Private practice and assorted pseudo-private activities—police surgeon work, occupational health, care home doctor, and so on—contribute only tiny amounts to the total economy of general practice, even if they do occasionally make significant differences to individual incomes. Practices have accounts and aim to make profits, which they disburse within themselves, but this does not make them into 'businesses', with all the implications of trading at a profit or loss and running the risk of business failure, any more than the accounts of a local branch of the Women's Institute make it into a commercial enterprise. Since 1948 GPs have not run any trading risk, their incomes being guaranteed by the NHS. Although it was possible for a practice to go bust between 1948 and recently, in reality it did not happen because somebody (new blood) or something (an NHS management body) intervened, either by turning its fortunes round or by dispersing its patients among neighbouring practices. The independent contractor status has mythical properties for general practice, but the contractual relationship we have with the State might be better seen as highly dependent. Most of us know this, which may be why when asked we attribute professional autonomy more to the absence of hierarchically deployed policies and incentives than to our employed or self-employed status.[6] Two points arise from this that will recur throughout this exploration of industrialization. The first is that words and ideas that are common currency can obscure real relationships. The second is that things that are more wishful thinking than real—the independent contractor status—may come into being as the old relationships between general practice and the NHS are changed. Independent businesses, in the sense of commercial groups open to competition and at risk of commercial failure, are appearing in and around general practice.

The form of economic organization that seems to describe best the position of general practice within the NHS is a combination of franchising (an external arrangement between the practice and the NHS) and co-operatives (an internal arrangement between those investing time and money in the practice). Franchises are alliances between large-scale, capital-rich organizations and small-scale entrepreneurs with experience, local expertise, and contacts.[7] The Franchisor lends its name (which it promotes) and to a variable extent its resources (subsidies for staff, free access to training, material goods such as computer hardware) to the Franchisee, in exchange for commitment to the Franchisor. The most important thing the Franchisor brings, however, is trading stability, with the potential to underwrite costs so that the risks of failure are greatly reduced. Franchisees hire and fire staff, provide services and are able to make profits. They can sell burgers, car exhausts, or mobile phones. Franchises can grow quickly, utilizing the local knowledge and energy of entrepreneurs whose risks are reduced by the franchisor, and are a formidable way of organizing service industries. The NHS was able to create a nation-wide network of primary care services literally overnight in 1948 by organizing a franchise arrangement with existing professionals who no longer had to struggle against each other in competition for patients. The relative autonomy of franchisees that GPs experienced between 1948 and 1990 did not mean that they were not part of the NHS 'industry', but it did mean that they were not directly controlled, on a day-to-day basis. Their relationship to the health service was an arms' length one.

However, there can be disadvantages to franchises, because once their range of services expands they have problems maintaining the quality and consistency of their activity, and this encourages the Franchisor to take direct control of the local service outlet. There was, therefore, already a potential for incorporation of general practice into the main structure of the NHS industry from the outset. If the scope and scale of general practice increased to incorporate a wider range of clinical activities strains would appear in the trading relationship, particularly if practice development were uneven and the quality of care inconsistent.

Co-operatives require their memberships to invest in the enterprise, and share the gains or losses. The co-operative way of working is a powerful way of involving individuals in group effort. Its disadvantage is that co-operatives can be more conservative in their investment decisions than types of economic organization that are more accustomed to taking financial risks. One very prominent example of this is the story of the Langwith village surgery, where North East Derbyshire PCT had decided to transfer control of an underperforming service to a multinational corporation, United Health Europe, before being halted by a crusading local GP, Elizabeth Barrett. The story was presented as a David and Goliath struggle by the medical press, with a happy antiprivatization ending in which the village surgery remained within the NHS under new leadership.[8,9] This version is not wrong, but the story can be told with different emphases. The Langwith village surgery had been offered to the Shirebrook practice, where Dr Barrett worked, but the practice had decided that it did not have the capacity to absorb it. Elizabeth Barrett's own words about the conflict vindicate the belief that market mechanisms can mobilize professionals who are otherwise unwilling to take on extra tasks and challenges: 'The process has totally changed me—it has been an explosive and exponential learning curve. I have always been a conformist, but as I get older I realise … it doesn't matter much if I upset a few apple carts.'[8] The second differing emphasis is similar, if less obviously transformative: the village surgery had been run, unsuccessfully, as a nurse-led unit, which had attracted a lot of complaints. We shall see the significance of this more clearly in the chapter on Forward Integration.

Public domain and public sector

The franchise arrangement between the NHS and general practice placed the discipline firmly in the *public domain* without incorporating it formally into the *public sector*. David Marquand describes the public function of allegedly independent professionals like this:

> Doctors … are not rationally calculating market actors, behaving in accordance with the profit motive—or, at any rate, not solely. At least in principle they are supposed to abide by an ethic of public service that tells them to pursue the public interest, even if they earn their living in a market of some sort.

They are not agents of their clients alone. They are also the agents of the public at large. Of course, they may fail to discharge their public service obligations, but if they do so they dishonour their vocation.[10]

He goes on to argue three propositions. First, that the public domain is a mechanism by which markets are mastered for the public good. Second, that professionals such as GPs are therefore fundamentally antimarket. Third, that the definition of the public good is not fixed but inherently contestable, and made through conflict and the resolution of conflict. According to Marquand, the definition of professionalism also shifts, starting out in the period around the Second World War (when the NHS was conceived) as a commitment to the public good and evolving (just as Raymond Williams described) to mean the possession of knowledge, technical skills,, and qualifications that the public lacked. These two themes, the public domain and the contestability of the 'public good', will appear in different forms throughout this account of the industrialization of general practice.

The franchise and the co-operative bring local knowledge and expertise to bear on local economies. This fitted well with the gatekeeper role of general practice, when the primary function of the GP was to sort out those who needed specialist assessment and treatment from those who did not. This was and still is a substantial task. A quarter or more of those visiting their GPs are likely to have sufficient recurring difficulties with work and relationships to meet the criteria for personality disorder.[11] Somatization of distress into packages of physical symptoms is widespread, even if the full psychiatric category of somatization disorder is uncommon, and reattributing symptoms to causes is a difficult job. As we all respond differently to challenges to our health, according to gender, family tradition, wealth or deprivation, insider or outside status and other pressures, general practice requires a wide understanding of the effects of culture on health and illness. Knowing about the characteristics of the local population— such as the imminent loss of jobs in a dominant industry, recent migration into the UK, pockets of long-term poverty—as well what makes individuality—the dynamics of families, explanatory models of health and illness, self-efficacy and help-seeking behaviour— matters in general practice because they are the basis for smarter gatekeeping.

Industrialization begins: the 1990 contract

The qualities of the franchise and the co-operative were tested in the first phase of industrialization, the turbulent period of change between 1990 and 1999. The franchise system became strained as general practice accumulated public health functions (immunization, cervical cytology screening, and provision of contraceptive services) and began to produce the variations in the quantity and quality of care that with hindsight seem inevitable given the lose managerial relationship of general practice to the NHS. One immediate consequence was that the centralizing potential inherent within franchising became attractive to the health service's management. The Department of Health, unable to reach agreement with the profession, imposed a much 'tighter' contract on general practice. The 1990 contract substantially reduced clinical autonomy by introducing detailed contractual duties such as 3-yearly health checks for adults, annual check for older patients, and production of annual reports, and also by constraining prescribing through the introduction of limited lists and indicative drug budgets.[12] The lack of scientific evidence of benefit from 'health checks' (which were a red flag symptom of the consumerist mood in government) led rapidly to the abolition of those for working age adults, but the '75 and over checks' languished in the GP contract until 2004, unpoliced and largely unimplemented. The huge tensions that arose produced conflicts with the government around out-of-hours working and a desire to define 'core services' within general practice.[12] Rudolph Klein describes the political battles that occurred between the BMA and the Department of Health in detail, but the essence of the campaign waged by GPs was an attempt to restrict the 'product range' of services provided in order to retain some degree of autonomy over everyday clinical practice and the organization of time. The main beneficiaries of the 1990 contract were the practices that had anticipated change and expanded over the period 1988–92, restructuring their partnership organization and enhancing or adding the skills of a manager, but even then only a tiny minority (about 5%) maximized their remuneration under the new contract.[13] Nevertheless Rudolf Klein was able to note that 'GPs could find consolation in the fact that their defeat had been highly profitable: in the first year of the new contract their income exceeded the intended target by £6,000 a head. Militancy was doused by prosperity'.[14]

Market reforms

General practice was also caught up in changes in the wider health service, upon which it was almost completely dependent. These changes were driven by the view that the system of NHS hospitals was inefficient and that it could not provide value for taxpayers' money until its inefficiencies were extirpated. The disciplinary force that would banish inefficiencies was not bureaucracy—the ever-tighter management discipline that expressed itself in the 1990 GP contract—but the market. Health Authorities would purchase specialist care from hospitals, and the buying and selling would make hospital managers and clinicians more aware of costs (and the need to be efficient) and more responsive to customers, which in this situation were Health Authorities not patients. General practice could play a part in all this if practice adopted budgets and played the market too—the period of 'fundholding' began. The introduction of competitive discipline into the NHS hospital system through the construction of this so-called 'internal market' was meant to increase efficiency so much that the need for additional funding for the NHS could be avoided. This pre-occupation with cost containment revealed one of the fatal flaws of market thinking, the central importance of clinical effectiveness—the certainty that what is being purchased actually works—which is a prerequisite for efficiency. This problem was barely addressed by the 1991 reforms, which seemed to generate endless managerial debates about 'quality' but few about the effectiveness of health services. New ideas about evidence-based medicine and evidence-based practice were adopted by NHS managers as a way of restricting or reducing services, so maintaining the underlying focus on cost containment. Throughout the period of the internal market the NHS was managed according to cost and process criteria, not effectiveness or quality of care, and both the Department of Health and the market, such as it was, failed to define, measure, and implement quality outcome policies.[15] As we shall see later in the discussion of fundholding, GPs were on the sidelines of these debates about cost, because they were focused on issues of access to specialist services, through reduced waiting times, specialist outreach clinics, or in-house physiotherapy. This interest in time and location as two aspects of service quality meant that GPs with impeccable antimarket credentials could engage with the fundholding process.

There was at the time an alternative approach to NHS reform, also designed to achieve high quality healthcare while containing costs, which was based on the widespread promotion of effectiveness, rather than competition, as the stimulus to improved quality and efficiency.[16] Its author, the American Louise Quam, argued that clinical effectiveness is a prerequisite for 'value for money', whatever the system of financing, but also that the market reforms made the possibilities for the successful promotion of clinical effectiveness *less* likely than before, because of the short-term thinking, fragmentation of services, and secrecy about investment plans that would result from the introduction of market mechanisms. This view prevailed in the second phase of industrialization, after 1999.

In keeping with the government's desire both to control the costs of healthcare and to promote increased choice for 'consumers', two distinct and wholly incompatible market structures were created, both of immediate significance for general practice.. These differed by virtue of the characteristics of the purchaser of healthcare, and have been termed type I and type II markets.[17] In both, the providers of care are public sector hospitals and community services, as well as commercial and voluntary sector organizations.

The type I market is based on a 'needs-led' model of healthcare purchasing and is sometimes called an 'industrial' market. In this market, the purchaser is a health authority, acting on behalf of a geographically defined, resident population. The basis for purchasing decisions is the utilitarian one of maximizing the 'health gain', which can be achieved for the population as a whole from a fixed budget. The authority is charged with the responsibility of undertaking 'health needs assessments' to determine both the state of health of its population and the services that are required to meet the needs so identified. This process requires evidence on the effectiveness and cost-effectiveness of all possible interventions, so as to maximize the potential health gain that can be achieved.

By contrast, the type II market (sometimes called a 'retail' market) is based on a 'demand-led' model. Here, the market existed between providers and those GPs who had chosen to hold their own budget for hospital and community care, the fundholders. The characteristics of the GP purchaser were quite different from those of the health authority. There was no requirement to assess the health needs of a population, nor even necessarily of the list of enrolled patients, but only to respond to individual demand as it presented itself in the consulting room with an eye to its impact on the budget. Nor was there any requirement to assess the likely effectiveness of different possible strategies for prevention and treatment, but only, ultimately, to act as an agent for the individual patient in arranging for care that will meet their needs and satisfy their preferences. However, since the 1990 contract had created a range of public health tasks for GPs that did depend on some assessment of need, such as the '75 and over checks', this superimposition of a retail market function put GPs in the position of having to play two different, and potentially contradictory, roles simultaneously. We will return to the impact this had on GPs themselves later in this chapter.

Patients as customers

In the type II market there was also the possibility that individuals might choose to change GP on the basis of their fundholding status or purchasing policies. Similarly, GPs could in theory have chosen to remove patients from their lists or refuse to accept new patients if they look as if they will be heavy users of the fund. The devolution of budgets to primary care physicians, in the form of GP fundholding, therefore created not only a market between fundholders and hospitals—a provider market—but also the possibility of market-like behaviour between patients and their GPs—a purchaser market, in which patients really could become customers. Such a development was encouraged by the liberalization of practice advertising and by simplifying the procedures for changing doctors, and would be expected to lead to increasingly overt competition between fundholders for patients—and particularly, of course, for those patients least likely to need care. In the event, little purchaser competition emerged.

Mullen described the confusion that accompanied the policy-making debate over the NHS reforms, as these two distinct market structures were created without any clear understanding of their quite different implications for efficiency, equity, choice, and cost control.[17] The type I (health authority) model allowed a high degree of control over both costs and the ability to promote priorities for healthcare expenditure. Health authorities purchasing for defined populations are able, at least potentially, to identify and address public health priorities, the interests of different population groups, the possibility of unmet (and perhaps unexpressed) need, and the promotion of equity of access to healthcare. However, this strong population perspective comes at the price of freedom of choice for patients and their GPs, who are supposed to keep within the bounds of the contracts agreed on their behalf by the planners. The autonomy of the GP becomes increasingly constrained as the health authority applies increasingly complex and stringent rules about what services could be used, what medicines should be prescribed, and what GPs themselves might do.

The type II (fundholder) model allowed far greater freedom of choice to GPs and, in theory, to patients. Practices could negotiate for acute and community trusts to provide them with services that are cheaper, quicker or more convenient than previously, without the layers of bureaucracy entailed by health authority purchasing. The other side of this coin was that, while emphasizing responsiveness to patients, practices have no need to consider the community beyond their list (although many fundholders actually did). Not only is the rationale for purchasing quite different, but the population covered is so small that, for anything but the most common conditions, the demand for services will fluctuate wildly from year to year.

Two versions of the public good

The two purchasers of the NHS and their respective markets soon came to represent the competing political ideologies driving British healthcare reform. On the one hand, the health authority embodied the rational planning instincts of those seeking to contain healthcare costs and maximize efficiency in the use of resources, and on the other

GP fundholders embodied the aspirations of those who would achieve efficiency—and consumer choice—through the promotion of as free a market as politically possible. The tensions evident in the objectives of reform were carried through into the structures designed to sustain the reform, in particular within the management of the health service. Far from creating a system in which bureaucracy melted away, providers freely competed for business and patients were always respected, the post-reform NHS generated new battalions of managers, new layers of regulatory control and a fragmented service in which patients remained confused and powerless. As we shall see later, this expansion of the managerial workforce had a more lasting effect on general practice than the contradictory demands of the NHS.

The reforms were intended to secure increased efficiency through competition between providers in a market in which, as in any shopping street, prices are published and are visible to all the players in the system. Indeed, it was explicit Department of Health policy that providers should make public their tariffs to encourage such competition. The picture painted at the outset of the reforms was of a market in which purchasers—health authorities and fundholders alike—would 'shop around' for the cheapest, quickest, or best quality care.

In reality the NHS internal market had none of the characteristics of a retail market, and stubbornly refused to behave like one.[18] It had much more in common with an 'industrial market', in which there are few purchasers and providers, the product is complex and infinitely variable and providers carry a high proportion of fixed costs. The result was that packages of care—and prices—were negotiated privately between purchasers and providers, and relationships tended to be long term. In itself this was not necessarily harmful to the efficiency of the market. In practice, though, the lack of fixed and observable prices rendered impossible the health authority's theoretical task of maximizing the 'health gain' achievable from limited resources.

The impact of the quasi-market in the NHS was minimal,[19] partly because of the retention of central government control and partly because the experiment was based on inadequate understanding of professional and managerial motivations.[20] Market mechanisms function differently in different healthcare structures. In Britain's system of 'hierarchical corporatism' accommodations between professional bodies and State institutions temper the pace of change, while turbulent transformation is a feature of the US healthcare system.[21] For example, competition in the supply of hospital services had only a limited impact on prices of specialist care, with high levels of variability in prices, widespread disregard for pricing rules and only some indications that GP fundholders were offered lower prices.[22] Economic evaluation appeared to play little part in decision-making, partly because of concerns about the validity of economic studies but also because multiple objectives were being pursued, increased efficiency being only one.[23]

There are other good reasons to suppose that the market, even had it 'matured', would not have behaved as planned. For example, as health authorities moved away from simple block contracting and towards more specific contracting arrangements, the challenge of negotiating contracts that balanced the financial incentives for providers with the desire of the health authority to get the maximum from its resources became ever more difficult. Agree too high a price, or for too many patients, and the purchaser wastes public money. Too low a price, or for too few patients, and hospitals lower their quality standards or stop treating patients before the year end. Set the contract for too short a period (and many managers argued that one year was too short) and risk perverse incentives for hospitals to underperform. Set the contract for a longer period, and lose the supposed benefits of competitive contracting as hospitals allow quality to slip or costs to rise.

Managed competition

It would have been difficult enough if it really were a competitive market. But at the same time as establishing radical new structures intended to encourage competitive behaviour, the NHS Executive drew the lines of regulation and monitoring so tightly that no real competition was allowed to emerge. Of course, in very many parts of the country competition was always wholly unrealistic because providers, especially community services, were effectively local monopolies. Yet even in London and other large cities that might actually have been able to support a competitive provider market, regulation was been as tight—or tighter—than anywhere else. The NHS Executive constantly intervened to impose or refuse mergers between providers, to prevent health authorities from moving their contracts away from underperforming hospitals that might become non-viable as a result,[24] to regulate capital borrowing by trusts and to disallow cross-subsidies between services within the same provider. Indeed, in some districts with two or more large providers, health authorities came to local agreements with hospitals designating each as the 'lead provider' in particular services, effectively neutralizing any possibility of competition.

Market theorists moved from straightforward competition to the notion of 'contestability' as a way of resolving this problem.[25] It may be enough just to have the threat of competition, they argued, for providers to improve their performance. While this may be true so long as the threat seems real, one could not continue to use 'contestability' as a policy instrument if the threat was never likely to become reality. The idea of contestability is weakened further by the observation that the high level of start-up investment required poses a significant barrier to new providers entering the healthcare market. In many places, even contestability was unrealistic.

The picture of 'managed competition' which emerged in the post-1991 NHS was one in which management heavily outweighed competition. While the Department of Health continued to talk in terms of 'the process of devolution stimulated by the NHS reforms', the reality was that political and managerial power in the health service became more centralized,[26] a trend consolidated by the transformation of the former regional health authorities into the arms of the Department of Health. One political commentator described the outcome of the reforms as 'neo-nationalization'.[27]

Given such developments, it is natural to ask whether the supposed benefits of competition could possibly emerge from a market in which almost no competition seemed actually to exist. The government seemed to have created a system in which it was paying for all the costs of competition—which included fragmentation, confusion, perverse incentives and erosion of a public service ethic, as well as the purely financial costs—yet was getting none of the benefits. This was clearly a disastrous waste of time and resources that had to be rectified, but before we examine how this was done in the second phase of industrialization, I want to return to fundholding as a way of working in general practice.

Fundholding revisited

Engagement of British GPs in market reforms through fundholding (1991–99) produced much political conflict but remarkably little benefit to the health of the population. It did, however, demonstrate how GPs perceived their role within the NHS, and the extent to which they were engaged in the modernization of the health service. Fundholders were expected to promote competition between hospitals for their custom, and this market was expected to function as a retail (type II) market.[17] The successes of some fundholders in creating a competitive environment led some analysts to overstate the impact of the move towards a market-based NHS,[28] for the evidence suggests that the overall impact of the marketization policy of this period on the organization and performance of GPs and hospitals was modest.[29,30] Fundholding appeared to promote greater inequality between practices and reduced the capacity of the NHS to plan strategically.[31] It achieved some cost savings in prescribing, but not in referrals to specialist care, and incurred substantial additional administration and transaction costs without demonstrating any improvement in health outcomes, nor any widening of consumer choice.[32]

While a few GPs embraced the concept of fundholding with enthusiasm at the outset,[33] there was widespread concern about the possible adverse effects for practices and patients, including fears that equity of access to services would be undermined and that the administrative structures required would become a considerable extra burden. However, a combination of pressure from the Family Health Service Authorities and GP investment in management skills and information technology drew an increasing number of GPs towards fundholding. This enrolment could not alter the contradictoriness of the whole market approach, so despite the expansion of fundholding to cover 40% of the population by 1995, it soon became a policy problem for the then Conservative government. First hailed as a success,[34] it became dogged by limited advantages, high costs, and unintended consequences, of which perhaps the greatest was the perceived assault on equitable provision of healthcare.

The only area where fundholders showed a demonstrable advantage over non-fundholding GPs was in reducing prescribing costs.[35,36] This was a government objective, but success in cost containment tells us nothing about either the quality of care, which may decline as medicine costs are cut, nor the long-term economic costs of short-term savings on prescribing, which may be considerable.[37] As medication costs were being transferred to patients through higher prescription charges and a widening range of over-the-counter medicines, one possible end result of downward pressure on prescribing costs is greater expenditure on medication by those who can afford them, and less use of medication by those who cannot, a prospect that further reinforced fears about loss of equity.

The economic costs of fundholding were substantial, and included both open costs such as management fees, subsidies for computerization and administrative costs in the practice from the billing and contract review processes, as well as hidden costs such as staff time in Family Health Service Authorities, Trust hospitals, and the Audit Commission (a government agency that investigates the efficiency of public organizations). A number of estimates have been made of the additional administrative costs incurred by the fundholding scheme. Petchey calculated that the operating costs of fundholding in 1993–94 amounted to £66.6m or 3.5% of the total fundholding budget, and added that £165m was paid to fundholders between 1990 and 1995 for managerial support.[38] A survey carried out by *Fundholding* magazine suggested that the annual cost of managing fundholding might reach £80 000 per practice,[39] and even a riposte by two fundholders conceded a figure of about £60 000 was realistic.[40] It was clear that the transaction costs of fundholding were considerably higher than those of health authority commissioning. For example, Davies estimated practice-based management costs at about 6% of an average fundholder's practice budget. This contrasts with the management costs of a Health Authority, estimated to be about 1.7%.[41]

The opportunity costs of developing fundholding were not debated, but diverting resources to already well endowed suburban and rural practices to enhance their purchasing power while not spending development money on primary care services in deprived areas (outside London) was an assault on equity. The political costs were equally significant, given the damage done to equity by fundholders buying speedier treatment for their patients—'fast tracking'—which appeared impossible to prove but was accepted as fact whenever fundholders and trust business managers spoke off the record.

The demise of fundholding

For all these reasons fundholding failed as a mechanism for giving GPs leverage over specialist services, and was wound down between 1997 and 1999. It became so problematic for three reasons. First, fundholders usually could not act as ruthless purchasers. Not only is there a contradiction between the doctor acting in the patient's interest and the rationing of resources within a limited fund, but local providers (hospitals and community services) may not always be influenced by fundholders' interests, and choice of provider may be limited or non-existent.[41]

Second, fundholders were as much a threat as an opportunity for local health planning. Fundholders' decisions about placing resources were primarily budget-led because the pressure to avoid overspending was so great. Overspent fundholders simply lacked the money to pursue wider health policies, even if they wanted to. In addition, evidence emerged of ambivalence in purchasing community services (as opposed to acute hospital care),[42] an overwhelming focus on the development of in-house physiotherapy and counselling to the exclusion of other agendas, and the risk of fragmenting specialist services by establishing outreach clinics.[43]

Finally, general practice had already evolved beyond the gatekeeper role. The 1990 contract change confirmed and extended changes already underway, driven in part by the professional perspective of the Royal College of General Practitioners, and in part by public health specialists seeking a way to change the nation's health. No school of general practice saw itself as *only* having a gatekeeper function that controls access to specialist medicine, but fundholding stressed the over-riding importance of the prudent gatekeeper. The costs of specialist care may have been reduced by better chronic disease management in the community, and through primary and secondary prevention in general practice, but we still cannot be certain about that and the opposite could be true. Inadequate screening, health maintenance and disease management by cost-conscious general practices could create more downstream problems for specialists, requiring more money not less to solve them. A mechanism that encouraged less referral or prescribing on the assumption that other forms of treatment will then develop to make this reduction possible was running far ahead of the evidence.

This failure came about because fundholding developed as an ideological construct, not a scientific hypothesis. Fundholding was an idea that evolved from a micro-economic model of general practice development[44] and was promoted by 'ignorant experts' (Alan Maynard, unpublished discussion paper) but never tested in pilot studies, despite authoritative advice from US market guru Einthoven that this should be done.[45] Designed as a political solution to 'kick start' the NHS internal market, fundholding became an end in itself.[46]

The impact on general practitioners

Two telling changes occurred within general practice in response to the tightening of the contract and the conflicts around fundholding. First, GP job satisfaction dropped after 1990/1 then slowly recovered as practices adapted to the changes imposed upon them, but did not return to 1987 levels even though income rose.[47] Dissatisfaction in 1990 increased for the rate of pay, the hours of work, the opportunity to utilize abilities, job variety, the amount of responsibility, and choice of ways of working. It remained unchanged against 1987 with the physical environment and with colleagues and fellow workers. Clinical autonomy, it seemed, was more important for doctors than managerial autonomy,[48] and was perceived as being under threat from the 1990 reforms and the introduction of market mechanisms in 1991. Autonomy—the ability to control at least some aspects of the working day—declines as the identity of the worker becomes submerged in the overall division of labour, with the result that the worker becomes alienated and de-skilled, and disinvests psychologically from the work.[49]

Second, larger practices developed management structures that permitted managers to delegate tasks more often, and take on a more strategic and executive role.[50] Not only did this development show the adaptability of general practice, but it signalled the entry of management into the work unit. Running the practice was no longer an administrative task for the senior partner's spouse.

The rise of management

If one aim of the market reforms of 1991 was to reduce NHS bureaucracy, on this count alone they would have to be judged a spectacular failure. Inevitably, the information and accounting tasks associated with the introduction of a market resulted in an enormous increase in the number of health service managers and administrative and clerical staff. The most public and therefore most controversial expression of the cost of the market has been in the almost exponential rise in health service managers. Between 1988 and 1993 the number of general and senior managers rose from 1240 to 20 010.[51] Public concern over this apparently burgeoning bureaucracy prompted repeated government protestations that much of the increase could be explained in terms of the reclassification of nursing and administrative posts as managerial ones. None the less, there was no denying that a large proportion of the increase was a genuine expansion in managerial numbers, estimated by one analyst as an additional 1700 managers over the period 1991–94.[52]

All of these additional costs that resulted (at least in part) from the creation of the internal market posed an important, and as yet unanswered, challenge to the claim that the reforms secured 'best value for money'. It is at least possible that the old, bureaucratic way of doing things was, in fact, more efficient after all. Some theoretical support for this idea comes from the work of the economist Oliver Williamson, who examined the conditions under which management hierarchies are more efficient than market relationships (discussed in Robinson and Le Grand[25]). In the light of this, it is arguable that the characteristics of healthcare provision are such that the attempt to replace hierarchical with market-like structures will lead to a fall in efficiency. This awareness fuelled by the obvious failure of the type II market experiment and the discontent within the medical profession, led the new government of 1997 to shift the emphasis back towards hierarchical management but without entirely dropping the use of market discipline. The day of the type I market had arrived, and the second phase of the industrialization of general practice began.

Enter primary care groups

In the phase of reforms introduced in 1997, general practice became further incorporated into health service management through the formation of Primary Care Groups (PCGs) and Trusts (PCTs), which in effect began to collectivize previously semi-autonomous practitioners. This swing back towards a social rather than market model still contained features from the earlier market orientation, which are discussed elsewhere.[53] The economic structure that was created was more of an industrial market (type I market) than a retail one, with supportive rather than competitive relationships between healthcare providers. The primary care groups required GPs and primary care teams to improve the health of their communities by addressing the health needs of their population, promote the health of that population and work with other organizations to deliver effective and appropriate care.[54] The potential problems of this approach included the negative effect of compulsory enrolling of reluctant GPs,[55] and the wide variations in prescribing and referral that would come to complicate the rationalization of PCG/PCT funding.[56] The tendency of the NHS to undervalue the motivation of practitioners and overvalue sanctions[57] created the risk that the whole process of change would degenerate into a bureaucratic 'name and shame' culture.[58] One important issue in the development of PCGs and PCTs was the extent to which professionals could fend off managerial control of clinical decision-making. Although this erosion of clinical autonomy was anticipated, there was at the beginning of the change to a more planned economy of primary care little evidence that the new policies and management structures made much impression on clinical autonomy.[59] Just as fundholding appeared to be more inequitable than it actually was, so the formation of PCGs threatened autonomy more than they actually compromised it.

The effect of the threat to autonomy was significant and followed the pattern seen in 1990/1; GP job satisfaction fell between 1998 and 2001, but then recovered.[60] Job satisfaction is a weighty matter, with serious implications for health. An illuminating contemporaneous study of GP job satisfaction in Leeds suggested high levels of psychological symptoms, and perceived poor physical health among GPs, before the introduction of Out-of-Hours co-operatives.[52,61] This study should alert us to the health risks associated with the industrialization process. Imbalance between effort and reward is common among professionals, especially those working with large numbers of clients, and creates a state of emotional distress, autonomic arousal and physical strain effects,[62] particularly coronary heart disease.[63] Such imbalances are a feature of service jobs involving 'emotional labour', in which feelings are induced or suppressed to maintain an outward appearance that promotes a calm, stable, or otherwise functional state of mind in others.[64] Where job demands are high, and characterized by conflicts over time and behaviour, as well as by reduced capacity to control the work process, the adverse effects appear as hypertension, heart disease, fatigue, anxiety, and depression.[65] The response of GPs to early changes in the second phase of industrialization was to trade off one aspect of the new arrangements against another, to maximize autonomy. For example, a survey of GPs just prior to the implementation of the 2004 new General Medical Services (GMS) contract revealed support for those aspects of the contract that were perceived as reducing workload (such as shedding out-of-hours responsibilities) and enhancing salary, and opposition to those that increased targets and bureaucracy.[66] GPs disaffected by this process may have opted into salaried contracts, which may explain why their levels of job stress fell and their job satisfaction increased.[67]

The trade-offs that occurred around the 2004 new GMS contract are the substance of the following chapters, but before moving on to them I want to try and answer another question. If British general practice is changing its relationship to the wider health service, and becoming more closely integrated with health service planning while also adopting an expanded public health role, how is it likely to develop in the future? I think we need more than an awareness of the recent history of general practice to speculate about its future, because history does not repeat itself and it is too simple to believe that history contains lessons that can be learned. There are, of course, rules of thumb about the responses that our discipline makes to changes around it, but these are rules that apply to past events, and may be a poor guide to the future. What we can do is think about how industrialization affected others, to get some sense of the possibilities ahead of us. I want to explore the inner workings of industrialization further, using the example of professional engineers as a template.

Patterns of industrialization

The processes of industrialization elsewhere can be a useful way to think about the sometimes bewildering changes that have occurred in general practice. In the USA in the late nineteenth and early twentieth centuries the industrialization of engineering followed a pattern with a number of features[68] that may look familiar to practitioners who have attempted to adapt to contract changes, market mechanisms and the seemingly ceaseless reshuffling of the NHS management structure. There are five features.

1. **Internalization of market and price mechanisms, in the form of management.** Developing industries replaced the purchase of raw materials, labour, expertise, and distribution mechanisms in open markets with increasingly complex management structures that supervised acquisition, production, and distribution of products. The general practice of Doctors Finlay and Cameron was a simpler job than ours because there were so few treatments available, and so few specialists who (surgeons apart) had limited skills beyond diagnosis. Consultations and therapies could be purchased, or bestowed charitably at the discretion of the clinicians, or somehow paid for by *ad hoc* arrangements with local government or through sickness funds and mutual societies, but there were few enough rules governing this exchange to require only minimal management. Once effective treatments appeared, imaging became available and the range of clinical responses expanded, the whole (increasingly costly) business of medical care needed ever more adjustment, regulation, and control.

In the NHS this management process spans the regulation of new technologies as well as the fixing of pharmaceutical prices, the imposition of tariffs for treatments as well as the codification of good medical practice and the adjudication of disputes with professionals or administrative bodies. In social insurance systems, such as those of Germany or France, larger administrative machines are needed to regulate professionals' claims for reimbursement, to negotiate the limits of treatment plans, to fix prices, and to police eligibility.

2. **Forward integration with a distribution network**. Part of the process of internalization of markets includes taking control, where necessary, of suppliers and distributors, to make them more responsive to the needs of the industry. Taken to its logical conclusion, this process would see pharmaceutical production, the surgical supply industry and all professional roles incorporated under one management structure, but not even the planned economies of Socialist Europe achieved this. The NHS leads the world, however, in the extent to which the front-line 'distributors' of medical care—GPs and their teams—are incorporated into the healthcare system's management structure, and also in the extent of price regulation with the pharmaceutical industry. The changes in GP contracts begun in 1990 and continued with the new GMS contract in 2004 can be seen as progressive forward integration of the whole process of care, drawing general practice deeper into the public domain and closer to the public sector.

3. **Adoption of large-batch, continuous-process technology**. Craft production is replaced by mass production, with an emphasis on output volume. The emphasis of the industry switches from tailoring responses to individuals, to applying the available resources to people whose problems, expectations, and needs could be aggregated into a small number of categories, according to resource availability. A crude example is the view that all GPs need to know about skin disorders is whether they are sensitive to Betnovate or not, but there is evidence from studies of responses to one of the largest healthcare user-groups, the older

population, to say that health and social care professionals frame need in terms of the service's capacity, not the individual's requirements.[58,69] Batched into types, people are easier for the system to count and to manage, so that GPs can monitor their own clinical treatment of conditions deemed important from both public health and cost perspectives as part of the Quality Outcomes Framework, while the Department of Health can estimate the costs of an outpatient follow-up for a hernia repair and contrast it with the cost of a visit to the GP, as if the content of the two encounters were actually interchangeable.

4. **The application of Taylorist** (efficient working practices) **and Fordist** (production line) **approaches** in management, the design of production sites and the organization of the production processes. These are characterized by six activities:

   (a) *The central codification of knowledge.* The philosophy of this, applied to healthcare, is expressed in evidence-based medicine, and the practical application of codified knowledge appears as guidelines. These guidelines, expressed as algorithms and used remotely by triage nurses employed by NHS Direct, can be used to route people with symptoms that concern them into different therapy options, from purchasing over-the-counter analgesics to presenting themselves at the A&E department.

   (b) *The standardization of tools.* The performance of clinicians is easier to measure if they all use the same rules to perform tasks, such as applying one particular depression rating scale to make (or exclude) a diagnosis of major depression.

   (c) *The subdivision of labour.* Patients may not 'need' to be seen by a GP, when a nurse could do the same task cheaper, and they may not 'need' to wait to see a specialist when a GP with special interests is available faster.

   (d) *Machines replace human skills.* Guidelines can be written in to the software of electronic medical records so that the monitoring of the quality of care can be done automatically, without any professional intervention or interpretation. Similarly, the therapy may be digitalized, so that self-help websites can be promoted in an effort to replace face-to face discussion, and cheaper on-line cognitive-behavioural therapy replaces the expensive counselling session.

(e) *Incentive payments*. The fees paid for items of service with individual payments were a kind of incentive to offer particular services (such as contraception advice) or carry out particular tasks (such as immunization), but also a reward for work done. These were discretionary, allowing the GP who did not think increasing income was worth the effort of form-filling and signature-gathering, to opt out of doing so. The recent expansion of the number of clinical domains attracting incentive payments, and their aggregation into populations of patients treated to a remunerable standard, is different in that much larger sums of money are attached to each clinical activity in a contract where incentive payments are no longer marginal to practice economies. Individualized incentives, such as smoking cessation interventions, may be used to engage practice nurses or pharmacists in new activities, or, such as influenza immunization, be deployed at local level to achieve local targets.

(f) *Faster work processes*. Time matters. Patients 'need' to be seen within 48 hours, urgent referrals where cancer is suspected must be seen within 2 weeks, NHS Direct advises some callers to seek medical attention within 4 hours, repeat prescriptions should be turned round in a day or two.

5. **The incorporation of science** into the industry occurs through two routes:

(a) *Linkage of scientists with business itself*. The involvement of doctors with the pharmaceutical industry is well-known and rightly perceived as problematic, but it is much more a phenomenon of specialist medicine than of general practice, aside from a few opportunities for GPs to engage in commercial drug trials. The industrial connection that involves general practice is in local management of the NHS, with clinicians taking on management functions on PCGs and PCTs, becoming 'champions' of particular clinical tasks, or taking up regulatory functions such as appraisal. As we shall see in later chapters, this is a minority activity, and part of the re-differentiation of GPs whose identities are shifting from being 'inner-city', 'rural', or 'single-handed' to 'managerial', 'entrepreneurial' or 'salaried'.

(b) *The development of a utopian ideology that emphasizes the benefits of the application of science to society*, in the form being promoted by the industry. This ideology must be 'clinical governance' with its hopes for professional engagement in the re-engineering and re-configuration of services so that they become fit-for-purpose and provide value for money. During the industrialization process GPs differentiate into three types: (i) a managerially inclined minority who become directly and sometimes deeply engaged in the industrialization process, as elements of a 'soft bureaucracy' (see Chapter 2); (ii) the majority who continue to work as best they can in changing circumstances, but whose job satisfaction levels fall with each change, only to rise again as compensatory mechanisms begin to operate; and (iii) a disaffected minority, which opts for salaried posts, or leaves general practice through early retirement or by other routes.

Using this model of industrialization as an analytic framework has two advantages. It explains the sometimes complex development of British general practice over time and suggests coherence in processes of change that can appear mysterious. It also explains the failure of the market reforms of 1991–99, which adopted models of development exactly opposite to those of classic industrialization. Instead of forward integration of distributors of medical care (GPs) and Fordist standardization of work processes the market reforms of 1991–7 emphasized the retail function of small-scale producers. Although there was an increase in administration in general practices, it was concerned with comparing prices, shopping round and invoicing, not the internalization of market mechanisms. The current reforms correspond much more closely to the industrialization model described, with incorporation of previously franchized

GPs into a more precisely described and tightly managed production process.

We have to realize that such development has not taken place in all industries, even in the USA and certainly not in mainland Europe, because it can be resisted by employers and entrepreneurs, it may work only in expanding economies, and it does not necessarily satisfy consumers or service users. Its critics are clear that the introduction of industrial processes into medicine may lead to the objectification of the citizen, and the application of simple linear solutions to complex, systemic problems in an impersonal, deskilled, rule-driven environment. These risks will resurface in the following chapters, where I will try to work out how substantial they really are.

References

1. Honigsbaum F. *The division in British Medicine: a history of the separation of general practice from hospital care 1911–1968*. Kogan Page, London, 1979.

2. Hurst JW. Reforming health care in seven European nations. *Health Affairs* 1991; **10**(3): 7–21.

3. Klein R. *The new politics of the NHS*. Longman, London (3rd edn) 1995, p 197.

4. Iliffe S. From general practice to primary care: developments in general practice 1980 to 1995 and beyond: Part 1. *Postgrad Med J* 1996; **72**: 201–6.

5. Iliffe S. From general practice to primary care: developments in general practice 1980 to 1995 and beyond: Part 2. *Postgrad Med J* 1996; **72**: 539–46.

6. Dowdswell G, Harrison S, Wright W. The early days of primary care groups: general practitioners perceptions. *Health, Social Care Community* 2002; **10**: 46–54.

7. Iliffe S. Thinking through a salaried service for general practice. *BMJ* 1992; **304**: 1456–7.

8. Robinson F. No private matter: taking the fight against commerce to the courts. *New Generalist* 2006; **4**(4): 58–61.

9. Arie S. Can GPs compete with big business? *BMJ* 2006; 1172.

10. Marquand D. *Decline of the public*. Cambridge: Polity Press, 2004, p. 30.

11. Moran P, Jenkins R, Tylee A, *et al*. The prevalence of personality disorder among UK primary care attenders. *Acta Psychiatr Scand* 2000; **102**: 52–7.

12. Warwicker T. Managerialism and the British GP: the GP as manager and managed. *J Manage Med* 1998; **12**(6): 331–48.

13. Lynch M. Financial incentives and primary care provision in Britain: do general practitioners maximise their income? *Dev Health Econ Public Policy* 1998; **6**: 191–210.

14. Klein R. *op cit* p. 203.

15. Maynard A. Competition and quality: rhetoric and reality *Int J Qual Health Care* 1998; **10**(5): 379–84.

16. Quam L. Improving clinical effectiveness in the NHS: an alternative to the white paper. *BMJ* 1989; **299**: 448–50.

17. Mullen P. *Health and the internal market: implications of the white paper.* Discussion paper No. 25. Birmingham: University of Birmingham Health Services Management Centre, 1989.

18. Dawson D. *Costs and prices in the internal market: markets vs the NHS Management Executive Guidelines.* Centre for Health Economics Discussion Paper No. 115. York: University of York, 1994.

19. Glennester H. Competition and quality in health care: the UK experience *Int J Qual Health Care* 1998; **10**(5): 403–10.

20. Le Grand J. Competition, co-operation or control? Tales from the British National Health Service. *Health Affairs* 1999; **18**(3): 27–39.

21. Tuohy CH. Dynamics of a changing health sphere: the United States, Britain and Canada *Health Affairs* 1999; **18**(3): 114–34.

22. Propper C, Soderlund N. Competition in the NHS internal market: an overview of its effects on hospital prices and costs. *Health Econ* 1998; **7**(3): 187–97.

23. Drummond M, Cooke J, Walley T. Economic evaluation under managed competition: evidence from the UK. *Soc Sci Med* 1997; **45**(4): 583–95.

24. Le Grand J. Internal market rules OK. *BMJ* 1994; **309**: 1596–7.

25. Robinson R, Le Grand J. Contracting and the purchaser-provider split. In *Implementing planned markets in health care: balancing social and economic responsibility.* Saltman RB and von Otter C (eds). Buckingham: Open University Press, 1995.

26. Paton C. Firm control. *Health Serv J* 1992; 102: 20–2.

27. Jenkins S. *Accountable to none: the Tory nationalisation of Britain.* London: Hamish Hamilton, 1995.

28. Audit Commission. *What the doctor ordered.* London: HMSO, 1996.

29. Raferty J, Stevens A. Day case surgery trends in England: the influences of target setting and of general practitioner fundholding. *J Health Ser Res Policy* 1998; 3: 149–52.

30. Mays N, Mulligan J-A, Goodwin N. The British quasi-market in health care: a balance sheet of the evidence. *J Health Serv Res Policy*, 2000; **5**: 49–58.

31. Koperski M, Rodnick JE. Recent developments in primary care in the United Kingdom: from competition to community-oriented primary care. *J Fam Pract* 1999; **48**: 140–5.

32. Smith R, Wilton P. General practice fundholding: progress to date. *Br J Gen Pract* 1998; **48**: 1253–7.

33. Houghton K. Peak practices. *Health Serv J* 1993; **103**: 26–7.

34. Glennerster H, Owens P, Matsaganis M. *A foothold for fundholding.* London: Kings Fund Institute, 1992.

35. Bradlow J, Coulter A. Effect of fundholding and indicative prescribing schemes on general practitioners' prescribing costs. *BMJ* 1993; **307**: 1186–9.

36. Maxwell M, Heaney D, Howie JGR, Noble S. General practice fundholding: observations on prescribing patterns and costs using the defined daily dose method. *BMJ* 1993; **307**: 1190–4.

37. Teeling-Smith G. The economics of prescribing and under-prescribing. In *Medicines: responsible prescribing*. Wells FO (ed.). Queen's University Belfast, 1992.

38. Petchey R. General practitioner fundholding: weighing the evidence. *Lancet* 1995; **346**: 1139–42.

39. Davies J. How much does the scheme cost? *Fundholding* 1995; **4**(2): 22–4.

40. Morris R, Armstrong M. Do not overestimate the scheme's costs. *Fundholding* 1995; **4**(4): 13.

41. Freudenstein U. Fundholding from the inside. *Med World* 1993; **13**: 10–11.

42. Williams G, Flynn R, Pickard S. Paradoxes of GP fundholding: contracting for community health services in the British National Health Service. *Soc Sci Med* 1997; **45**(11): 1669–78.

43. Corney RH, Kerrison S. Fundholding in South Thames Region. *Br J Gen Pract* 1997; **47**(422): 553–6.

44. Bosanquet N, Leese B. *Family doctors and economic incentives*. Dartmouth: Aldershot, 1989.

45. Smith R. Words from the source: an interview with Alain Enthoven. *BMJ* 1989; **298**: 1166–8.

46. Willis A. Who needs fundholding? *Health Serv J* 1992; **102**: 24–5.

47. Sibbald B, Enzer I, Cooper C, Rout U, Sutherland V. GP job satisfaction in 1987, 1990 and 1990: lessons for the future? *Fam Pract* 2000; **17**: 364–71.

48. Lichtenstein RL. The job satisfaction and retention of physicians in organised settings: a literature review. *Med Care* 1998; **41**: 139–79.

49. Muntaner C, Benach J, Hadden W, Gimeno D, Benavides F. A glossary for the social epidemiology of work: part 2. Terms from the sociology of work and organisations. *J Epidemiol Community Health* 2006; **60**: 1010–12.

50. Westland M, Grimshaw J, Maitland J, Campbell M, Ledingham E, McLeod E. Understanding practice management: a qualitative study in practice management *J Manage Med* 1996; **10**(5): 29–37.

51. Department of Health. *Statistical Bulletin* 1994/11. HMSO.

52. Appleby J. Managers: in the ascendancy? *Health Serv J*, 1995; 32–3.

53. Iliffe S, Munro J. New Labour And Britain's National Health Service: an overview of current reforms. *Int J Health Serv* 2000; **30**: 309–34.

54. HSC 1998/228. *The new NHS modern and dependable primary care groups: delivering the agenda*. Leeds: Department of Health, 1998.

55. Smith R. What is a primary care group and how will it work? In *Evidence-based medicine: its relevance and application to primary care commissioning*.

Harrison S (ed.). Round table Series 59. London: Royal Society of Medicine Press, 1998.

56. Majeed A. Equity in the allocation of resources to general practice will be difficult to achieve. *BMJ* 1998; **316**: 43.

57. Ham C. Improving NHS performance: human behaviour and health policy. *BMJ* 1999; **319**: 1490–2.

58. Anon. *Clinical governance: from rhetoric to reality*. London: Thames Region NHSE, 1998.

59. Locock L, Regan E, Goodwin N. Managing or managed? Experiences of general practitioners in English Primary Care Groups and Trusts. *Health Serv Manage Res* 2004; **17**: 24–35.

60. Whalley D, Bojke C, Gravelle H, Sibbald B. GP job satisfaction in view of contract reform: a national survey. *Br J Gen Pract* 2006; **56**: 87–92.

61. Appleton K, House A, Dowell A. A survey of job satisfaction, sources of stress and psychological symptoms amoing general practitioners in Leeds. *Br J Gen Pract* 1998; **48**: 1059–63.

62. Siegrist J. Adverse effects of high-effort low reward conditions at work. *J Occup Health Psychol* 1996; **1**: 27–43.

63. Bosma H, Peter R, Siegrist J, *et al.* Two alternative job stress models and the risk of coronary heart disease. *Am J Public Health* 1998; **88**: 68–74.

64. Muntaner C, Benach J, Hadden W, Gimeno D, Benavides F. A glossary for the social epidemiology of work organisation: Part 1, Terms from social psychology. *J Epidemiol Community Health* 2006; **60**: 914–16.

65. Van der Doef M, Maes S. The job demand-control (-support) model and psychological well-being: a review of 20 years of empirical research. *Work Stress* 1999; **13**: 87–114.

66. Spurgeon P, Hicks C, Field S, Barwell F. The new GMS contract: impact and implications for managing the changes. *Health Serv Manage Res* 2005; **18**(2): 75–85.

67. Gosden T, Williams J, Petchey R, Leese B, Sibbald B. Salaried contracts in UK general practice: a study of job satisfaction and stress. *J Health Serv Res Policy* 2002.

68. Chant C (ed.). *Science, technology and everyday life 1870–1950*. London: Routledge, 1989.

69. Chevannes M. Social construction of the managerialism of needs assessment by health and social care professionals. *Health Soc Care Community* 2002; **10**(3): 168–78.

Chapter 2

General practice, management, and bureaucracy

Having no bureaucrats in general practice is what
keeps us efficient and stops us doing the silly
wasteful mistakes that are endemic in the NHS.
Dr Gwion Rhys, Nefyn, Gwynedd, The Guardian
(Monday 22 January 2007)

This last sentence in a letter to *The Guardian* about the excessively
high incomes of general practitioners (GPs) will provoke different
responses from different professions. Some, such as those charged
with containing prescribing costs, might see general practice as prone
to wastefulness, or even open to silliness. Managers in Primary Care
Trusts (PCTs) struggling with the administration of (in)dependent
contractors, the commissioning of secondary care and the provision
of community services might point out how the word 'bureaucrat' is
used pejoratively, and unfairly. I want to emphasize something else,
an error of fact, the supposed absence of bureaucrats from general
practice. Not only are they present within general practice in increasing numbers, but increasingly GPs make up these numbers, and
bureaucratic thinking is entering the consciousness of practitioners
and shaping our everyday work. This chapter is about the bureaucra-
tization of general practice, using the word in a non-pejorative way to
describe how management imperatives and the demands of clinical
work are influencing each other.

At the start of the twenty-first century all health services in industrial
societies are a constantly expanding collection of activities, driven by

an evolving understanding of the causes and consequences of ill-health, by a deepening technical expertise and by a widening range of therapies delivered by a growing number of professionals and disciplines. Even in the least planned of healthcare systems, such as those of the USA or Germany, where individuals have to arrange or at least apply for some form of insurance, or pay out of pocket, or (in the American case) go without, there is a need to keep the system as a whole as rational as possible, and productive rather than counterproductive. Governments intervene to regulate market-driven systems of healthcare so that gaps in provision are closed, or at least narrowed, using Medicare and Medicaid budgets and systems in the USA and ensuring universal provision through the General Locality Sickness Insurance mechanism (Allgemeine Orts Krankenkasse—AOK) in Germany. Britain's health service is, for historical reasons, much more tightly controlled than many in Europe, and general practice has had a managerial function as a gatekeeper to specialist care since the foundation of the National Health Service (NHS) in 1948, in an informal compact with government against consumerism. When there were fewer specialists, who had fewer methods of investigation and treatment at their disposal, and therefore did fewer things, this gatekeeper task was difficult but manageable, with ample opportunities for covert rationing of services.

Now there are more things that can be done by health professionals, and now that the population knows more about the possibilities of investigation and treatment, it is harder to control the gate against demand. We will return to the impact of consumerism in Chapter 7, but also need to recognize that a 'revolving door' effect may operate, in which the time and effort allocated to the management of long-term conditions such as diabetes and heart disease—very much part of the industrialization process—are taken away from meeting other demands in general practice (for example around common problems such as skin diseases and ENT complaints). One way to meet these seemingly lower-priority demands on time is to lower the threshold for seeking specialist help, a deliberate but not necessarily conscious relinquishment of the gatekeeper task. In addition, the emergence of newly recognized or constructed problems with protean characteristics, such as sleep apnoea, chronic fatigue syndrome, attention deficit hyperactivity disorder or mild cognitive impairment, makes the decision-making about opening the gate more and more difficult. The availability of imaging technologies makes achievement of certainty, or even maximal probability, increasingly possible and also increasingly problematic. It is not just the headache that might be a sign of a brain tumour that warrants an magnetic resonance imaging or computed tomography scan, but also the shoulder capsulitis and the knee injury that call for scanning. And the capacity to offer more or less effective treatments in general practice—obesity, Alzheimer's disease, schizophrenia—means that our decisions carry ever greater price tags. As the possibilities of medical care expand, the porousness of the barrier to specialist care that general practice once tried to provide increases. The autonomy of general practice, or rather its organizational distance from the management of specialist hospital care, which had been such a strength, is now becoming less effective as a solution, and is therefore becoming part of the problem.

The natural response from the Department of Health is to bring general practice inside the NHS management structure at least political and financial cost. The logic of this is that tighter control of what GPs actually do in their consultations seems a plausible way of strengthening the gatekeeper role. The problem for policy makers and managers is the political risk of being seen to control professional behaviour—to reduce autonomy—in a discipline with a long history of opposition to a salaried status for itself (at least until now). Autonomous practice and the kind of industrialized management favoured by the NHS are uncomfortable with each other, but the policy makers realize that some autonomy is desirable so that local issues are dealt with locally, and with discretion. The last thing that New Labour has wanted is the flight of the middle classes from the public health service into the commercial sector, so the local solution of the local problem—the tailoring of care to the individual—is something to be preserved. At the same time the price of medical care needs to be internalized within all clinical transactions, so that decision-making in general practice always takes into account both patient needs and system costs. A mechanism is needed, therefore, to make GPs increasingly concordant with clinical protocols, responsive to budget pressures within PCTs, and vulnerable to financial loss if they fail to satisfy both their patients and the NHS. The hunt is on, therefore, for a way of achieving objectives that seem to be contradictory. Or, to put it the other way round, the NHS management is seeking ways of making GPs better able to cope with the cognitive dissonance of their new and evolving situation.

Containing the tensions generated by contradictory objectives is difficult, but the NHS as an institution is creative, and policy makers are even more so. A flurry of initiatives appear, are tested and then fade away. Champions and change agents, Health Improvement Programmes (HImPs) and National Service Frameworks are launched with fanfares, are the talk of the NHS management for a while and then are relegated as new solutions are promoted. As a result primary care policy making appears messy and ragged, reflecting a process of 'disjointed incrementalism'.[1] Beneath the surface, however, are some general trends. Four processes have emerged from the efforts to constrain the organizational autonomy of general practice while preserving its engagement with individuals and localities. They are: finding the best configuration of local administration for the health service, enrolling a cadre of GPs in management, expanding management functions within practices, and engaging practices collectively in making investment decisions in local services—through practice-based commissioning (PBC).

Local administration

The sometimes bewildering changes in health service management, from Family Practitioner Committees to Family Health Services Authorities, then to Primary Care Groups (PCGs) and on to PCTs, are sometimes explained in the simplest and most cynical way. Unable to change the behaviour of professionals, governments keen to show how assiduous they are in addressing NHS problems just modify things under their control—the hapless health service bureaucracy. While there may be some truth in this, it is not the whole explanation. Striving after contradictory objectives requires a particular form of working with professionals, aptly called 'soft bureaucracy', which needs skills and alignments that need to be made and constantly renewed at local level. Everything depends on getting the managers with the right skills into the right place alongside the particular professionals in any given locality, if 'soft bureaucracy' is to work.

The manager's dilemma is: How can decentralized and flexible professional work organizations such as general practices be governed?[2] How can new rules be imposed on experienced clinicians whose professionalism is based on clinical autonomy and whose administrative relationship with the NHS has been based for 50 years on franchised autonomy? The solution appears to be the nurturing of a kind of self-governance that combines the new rules, imposed from outside, in return for some power to shape those rules, and their application at the local level. This is 'soft bureaucracy', a term popularized by Courpasson in his discussion of managerial approaches to domination, in 2000.[3]

'Soft bureaucracy' is not gentle, either for GPs or for PCT managers, because each party has to adjust to an unfamiliar way of working that may seem to contradict their previous experience, training, or orientation. The doctors have to surrender some autonomy over decision-making, perhaps at the level of which drugs they can prescribe but conceivably which specialists they can refer to, or even whether their referral if 'appropriate' or not. The managers have to renegotiate the amount of power that they cede to professionals, not just in principle (how many GPs are on the Professional Executive Committee) but in detail (exactly which drugs are prescribable). Chris Ham, Professor of Health Policy at the University of Birmingham, describes exactly how managers are to work with GPs:[4] 'The paradox of professional service organizations like …primary care practices is that they are staffed by a mix of innovators and conservatives. The stimulus of high quality managers is therefore essential in supporting the innovators and challenging the conservatives to improve care for patients'.

No one can claim to know best how to do this, and past experience provides as many negative lessons as positive. For example, GPs, practice nurses, and PCG managers had very different expectations of PCGs, which may not have been reconcilable, had PCGs with their proportionately large numbers of professionals in controlling positions, survived.[5]

Soft bureaucracy

For GPs the processes of 'soft bureaucracy' require the clear assignation of responsibility (especially where failure occurs), which often gets expressed as 'being accountable'. The demands to adopt new rules and standards are couched in professional terms of 'good practice' so that practitioners modify their behaviour to comply with the new rules. This change is offset, to some extent, by practitioner efforts to modify the rules or standards to allow some fuzziness about the definition of good practice. This can occur because of a trade-off between acceptance of new rules and recognition (by management) of special practitioner expertise, a trade-off that often takes the form of GPs taking up managerial functions or new clinical roles aligned to management objectives. We will return to medical managers in this chapter, and consider GPs with a special interest in Chapter 3.

None of this comes easily for general practice, and the NHS structure finds it hard too. Managers who have grown up in the command and control hierarchy of the NHS learned to wait for guidance and cascade information and demands downwards. The wiser ones realized that they had to negotiate flexibly with general practice, and could achieve some of their objectives that way with some practices some of the time. They could always direct blame for failure upwards—to the tier of management above that was unresponsive, unaware of their local problems, and too concerned with the needs of the Department of Health or the whims of Ministers—or downwards to the 'unprofessional' behaviour of GPs who would not change their ways. 'Soft bureaucracy' changes all this because managers are tasked to standardize the performance of primary care, and experience both highly specific job descriptions and appraisals that individualize success and failure.

Hunting for the optimal form of management means lots of change within the administrative machinery of the health service, and this change has to be driven by central government itself. A number of tensions arise within management because of this enforced decentralization and heightened accountability, and it is no surprise that early in the second phase of industrialization some PCGs regarded their Health Authorities as 'authoritarian',[6] as the old hard hierarchy turned into the new soft bureaucracy. Their experience seemed almost exactly the same as that of those GPs who described themselves as being 'kebabed' by the reforms of 1997 onwards.[7] The complexity of the tasks facing managers in PCGs is shown in a case study of four primary care organizations that identified the factors promoting innovation as inspired leadership, opportunities to learn, clinician input to management, timing of initiatives and their local adaptation, and external facilitation of change. Low morale was associated with the overwhelming pace of reform, inadequate staff experience and financial deficits.[8] Reorganizing the administrative structure does not necessarily help, as the old ways of working carry over into the new structures, producing a mixture of directive and facilitative management styles in PCTs.[9]

Because general practice is such demanding work we can easily forget (or not even notice) the huge anxieties within the management structure of the NHS. Tony McCaffrey, describing workshops with service managers, noted the ambiguities of their roles and the stress this caused them, their mistrust of their seniors, their feelings of powerlessness and their anticipation of defeat as the next round of change undid their work, and their almost purposeful isolation from each other and from the public.[10] It is possible that experienced problem-solvers, used to working in conditions of uncertainty and ambiguity, could alter the way in which management works. GPs engaged in PCT management may have effects that they do not anticipate. There is some evidence that movement of doctors into management changes both the doctors and the management. Clinical directors respond to their incorporation into management by creating new forms of expertise through assimilation, extending their jurisdiction within the organization in a process of re-professionalization.[11] GP newspaper displayed the banner headline 'Half of PCTs allow open-but-full lists' on the front page of its 19 January 2007 issue, reporting in the story below a spokesman from the Department of Health who said: 'The DoH position is crystal clear. Under the new contract GP lists are now either open or closed'. What is crystal clear at the top can be hazy below, especially if experienced GPs can explain the nuances of 'open-but-full' to sensible managers with other priorities.

Practice culture

The contradictory requirements that NHS managers have of primary care can be resolved, linguistically if not necessarily in terms of practitioner behaviour, by using the idea of 'practice culture'. Every practice, small or large, works in its own way, with different patterns of power relationships and ways of responding to internal and external pressures. These practice cultures do change, when seen through the eyes of NHS management, but the change can only be facilitated, not actively directed.[12] This view assumes that the accumulation of small cultural changes will lead to a qualitative change in the nature of general practice, although it is rarely clear how this will come about, or what it would actually be. Part of the task of middle management, therefore, is to buffer the demands of politicians and the capabilities and sensibilities of practitioners, modifying each as much as possible. There could not be a better expression of Unger's model of how change comes about.

The idea of practice culture has more than political use value for middle management. We use it too, to explain our responses to the outside world. One activity that occurs within organizations is sense-making, in which external events are noticed, appreciated according to their congruence with the beliefs held by individuals or the group, and acted upon. 'Each round of appreciation depends upon the outcome of previous rounds, and the action that occurs will shape what is noticed in the future'.[13] Collective identity—the culture of the practice—is created and reinforced by successive encounters with outside demands. This has immediate implications. As Kath Checkland and her colleagues point out,[13] discussion about 'barriers to change' within practices may underestimate the structural nature of resistance to change, which is not a barrier that is easily lifted, or even that is liftable at all. Resistance to change, especially when externally driven, may in fact be a central component of a practice's culture. For all of us this means that we can construct an explanation of why we are too busy to implement this or that new development, or make an investment that will bring rewards in the future, while still remaining in our own eyes good doctors who care about our patients.

An ideal approach to management of general practice from outside—in the form that GPs are now experiencing with the 2004 GMS contract—requires definition of performance criteria, development of indicators and methods of assessment, practice visits to collect data against these indicators and feedback of judgements to the practice.[14] The first two actions are carried out at national level, and the latter two are the functions of the local administration (currently the PCTs). There is a clear intention in this approach to stimulate change, using indicators not just as ways of measuring how much money practices should get but also as incentives to change practice, either by tightening up clinical activity to hit clinical targets such as optimal blood pressure control or influenza immunization, or by altering practice management to incorporate desirable activities, such as consultation with patients or concordance with employment law. This intention to engineer changes creates problems for both national standard-setters and local promoters of change, for both need to know which aspects of practice behaviour are important to change, which incentives produce the desired change and how best to balance a range of incentives packaged up in a contract. In other words, how do general practices change when they do?

Promoting change

The easy and banal answer is that practices differ so much that there will be different motivations to and mechanisms for change in different groups. The response to the incentives offered by the Quality and Outcomes Framework in the 2004 contract suggests the opposite, as the great majority of practices achieved high levels of performance very quickly, which could be interpreted as evidence of relative homogeneity in the culture of practice organization. This may be only part of the answer, however. We do not know if the responsiveness of general practices will be sustained or remain so uniform if the balance of incentives in the contract is modified. It is possible that the heterogeneity of practices—the very variability in performance and capability that was used as a justification for initiating an industrialization process with the 1990 contract—will re-appear as new standards and targets are introduced. This would fit with what we see around us, whenever we get chance to see how other practices work. We can reasonably argue that general practice can be either prone to inertia with change occurring infrequently, discontinuously and intentionally, or emergent and self-organizing in a state of constant, evolving and cumulative change.[15] Similarly, change may take place primarily within the organization that functions as an independent entity, or in response to pressures from outside. Triggers for change may be objectified goals with measured outcomes and clear feedback mechanisms—the classic audit cycle—or come about through pragmatic overlaps between individual interest and external demands, through conflicts within the group, or through a desire to promote changes in multiple aspects of practice activity and simply see what emerges.[16] Within these possibilities practice leaders (and managers) may set the rules of audit, encourage participation, interpret emerging change or take a strategic view of multiple agendas. Resistance to change can then be viewed in many ways as lack of clarity in setting goals, as differences between individual and organizational objectives, as part of the process of making sense of what is happening or as an inevitable and necessary feature of conflict.

This multiplicity of ways of changing (or avoiding change) must be a problem for any management structure that seeks to engineer the industrialization of independent contractor general practice into a cohesive and comprehensive system of primary care, especially when there is no reason to believe that practices have any fixed combination of characteristics. Organizations change as individual members come and go, and as members learn more about their own capacities and skills. The solution that the NHS administration has found, so far, is the easiest one that fits with the centralized nature of health service organization: a systems approach of measuring performance against standards. It is much easier to count the number of people with diabetes whose HbA1c levels are within the desirable range than to measure patient satisfaction reliably and robustly, and it is probably easier for clinicians to reduce HbA1c levels in a small number of people than to increase the satisfaction levels of an ever-changing and increasingly diverse population. This centrally-driven system of targets could dominate the industrialization process for some time, because the target domains could expand in number—the management of Parkinson's disease or of urinary incontinence, the identification of visual impairment or early functional decline in older people, or risk assessment of possible abuse of children could all be quantified, along with many other clinical problems—or deepen: watch out for natriuretic peptide measurement, or the use of Amsler grids.

However, two things may restrain the standard setters' enthusiasm for the easily countable. One may be GP resistance to an ever-widening tariff of targets, and the other will be the greater importance of other aspects of clinical work. There may come a point where the number of reminders popping up on the computer screen crowds out the practitioner's clinical attention to the individual patient, or the number of support staff dedicated to driving and documenting target achievement stretches the practice budget too far. Too much counting of what effective practices already do has been likened to driving through the rear-view mirror, analysing past success and immobilizing practice development in an obsolete model.[14] Performance indicators of the Quality and Outcomes Framework type may appear to offer quality improvements and reduced costs, but they may in fact deliver simplicity at the expense of meaning,[17] may be blunt, expensive, incomplete and distorting.[18] It is much harder to identify and incentivize the components of multidisciplinary working, public involvement in service development, nurse-led case management or the development of joint clinical directorates across general practice and specialist care. These changes require a futures-focused attitude that anticipates change and uses a values-driven style of management, with powerful clinical involvement. Such a shift in the industrialization process will need supporting in a different way, with a bottom-up rather than top-down style, and the balance of management could then shift towards encouraging continuous learning in practices. It would require the acceptance of variability between practices as useful and desirable within localities, as some take on tasks that meet the needs of whole populations—such as minor surgery, or hosting the rapid-access diagnostic clinic, or providing the base for child and family services.

Medical managers

For soft bureaucracy to work medical leadership must be incorporated into the industrialization process.[19] This cannot be tokenistic and advisory involvement, because the objective is the creation of a bridge between NHS management and clinical practice, creating shared ways of thinking and acting. Exactly how this is to be done is something that we shall return to in Chapter 6, but for the moment we should concentrate on the flexibilities are required of practitioners and mangers alike.

Richard Sennett has much to tell us about this flexibility. He argues that modern forms of flexibility contain three important elements:[20] (1) the discontinuous reinvention of institutions; (2) 'flexible specialization'; and (3) the concentration of power without centralization.

1. **Discontinuous reinvention of institutions**. Continuity and change get mixed up and muddled. The formation of PCGs was seen by some as a continuation of fund-holding by other means, but the formation of Care Trusts and the 'downsizing' and subsequent abolition of Health Authorities broke with the past structure and culture of the NHS. PBC, on the other hand, can be confused with fund-holding even though it is different from it in many ways.

2. **Flexible specialization**. This is 'Getting more varied products ever more quickly to market', according to Sennett (p. 51).[20] The HImP and NSF targets were the precursors to those of the 2004 GMS contract and all of them fit this description. Practices are expected to pick up new targets and adapt their everyday working styles to meet them, on a regular basis, with new targets appearing in waves. Is the intention to promote 'a strategy of permanent innovation: accommodation to ceaseless change, rather than an effort to control it'.[21] There is a sense in which general practice accommodates to the process of flexible specialization easily, because information (about patients and their individual congruence with target attainment) is readily accessible on computers, and can be modified and manipulated easily as targets change. Rapid decision-making is part of the work culture, and is consistent with small group work, and there is some willingness to let at least some of the shifting demands of the outside world determine what practitioners do. General practice as a discipline is responsive to patients to the extent that GPs will (albeit variably) think of alternative medicine as useful, despite its poor evidence base or even the lack of a plausible scientific rationale.

3. **Concentration of power without centralization.** Institutions are reorganized into fragments and nodes in a network, controlled by setting production targets that the work units can meet in any way that they think fit. This freedom is limited by their resources, and by targets that are difficult to achieve given their capabilities.[22] The result can be 'the managerial overburdening of small work groups with many diverse tasks.'[20] (p. 55). This description seems to fit both the overall reform underway in the NHS and the experience of those working in general practice. Abandoning a hierarchical structure with paternalistic or maternalistic styles of working can be a problem because blame for faults and failures can no longer be projected from one layer to another (lazy GPs, stupid Health Authority), but instead turns into a form of sibling rivalry, with projection of negative attributes to nearby groups, or growing interpersonal conflict between members of the same group.[23]

Sennett's warnings about the negative features of 'flexibility' should be noted, but also taken in context. One of the strengths of the franchise relationship is that it requires practitioners individually and in groups to manage local demands with locally appropriate methods, creating the practice cultures that soft bureaucracy seeks to co-opt and change. Practice management is a relatively new ingredient of practice culture, having expanded from small beginnings in the first phase of industrialization.

Practice management and the 'operating adhocracy'

Soft bureaucracy is a mechanism for managing the complexities and uncertainties that experts—such as GPs—deal with routinely on a daily basis, often in ways that are more implicit (flying on auto-pilot) than explicit. The traditional form of general practice is that of an 'operating adhocracy',[24] in which there is little standardization of knowledge, the emphasis is on problem-solving and practical 'know-how', and practitioners are expert and creative, but able to work in groups and to update their 'know-how' rapidly and frequently. Some external pressures to standardize knowledge do affect the operating adhocracy, such as the educational efforts of the Royal College of

General Practitioners, but these are not mandatory and it remains possible to work as a GP without being a member of the Royal College. While the RCGP's activities represent an attempt to create a professional bureaucracy that might influence, even one day direct, the performance of GPs, it is a weak attempt compared with that of, say, the Royal College of Physicians, which controls entry to specialist medicine, promotes audit of clinical practice, and shapes professional development.

Soft bureaucracy is an attempt to bring the operating adhocracy under the control of an administrative machine, which will codify knowledge, attempt to reduce variations and uncertainties in practice, and monitor performance against specified rules and targets. Practice management, which stands between the intentions of the soft bureaucracy of the PCT and the habits of the practitioners, has a lot to learn. One example of the hunger for management knowledge in practices was apparent in a report published by the Medical Defence Union in 2000, which described how 15 000 of its GP members (just under half the GP workforce) had requested its *significant event audit booklet* and 4000 practices in the UK had taken up its *risk management training programme* (over a third of all practices).[25]

Just as there are tensions between managers in PCTs and GPs, so too are there conflicts within practices between a new generation of practice managers who have a different perspective of what needs to be done from their employers. The new contract of 2004 defines the tasks of general practice in such detail that it represents a narrowing of strategic options for practices, which will force further changes on practice managers.[26] Practice managers struggled during the first phase of industrialization to adopt a strategic role in response to the external demands on practices. Kath Checkland gives seven reasons why they have found strategic functioning so difficult,[27] many of which seem to confirm the conservative stance towards investment inherent in the co-operative form of organization favoured by GPs:

1. Normative beliefs that all management responsibility lies with GPs.
2. Problems of authority—how far can managers go in thinking strategically?
3. Time constraints—too many administrative tasks, and a need for a different skill-mix.
4. Divisions between managerial and clinical work.

5. Failure of GPs to manage their managers.

6. Confusion about the legitimate role of the manager, even when there is an explicit job description.

7. Low morale, partly due to rapid NHS changes.

Strategic thinking is now essential at practice level, as the pace of industrialization accelerates. Any general practice that wishes to remain viable in a rapidly changing environment must carry out five functions,[28] as shown in Box 2.1.

Box 2.1 Five tasks for practice management: housekeeping and husbandry

1. *Provide services that address needs.* This is the core activity of general practice, and practitioners become expert in service provision, easily meeting simple targets and standards.

2. *Co-ordinate efforts within the organization.* This is the task of practice management, and leadership in co-ordination is likely to lie in part with managers and in part with at least some clinicians. However, it is a relatively underdeveloped area of expertise in practices, which until 1990 had only to respond to patient demand.

3. *Support and control the distribution of resources, the provision of training and the gathering and distribution of information about quality, costs, etc.* This has an administrative dimension but also a political one, in which rules about resource allocation (who goes on holiday and when) are developed, agreed and maintained (or revised).

4. *Forecast future needs, opportunities and threats, and compare internal capacity with external demand.* This is an area of thinking that has had to grow since 1990, and is enlarging to include commercial threats to general practice monopolies in some areas.

5. *Set long-term goals and objectives.* The increasing financial risks that general practices face will make strategic thinking increasingly important.

These functions will be needed beyond the practice as well as within it, if PBC becomes embedded as the dominant mechanism for shaping specialist services for local communities.

Practice-based commissioning

Practice Based Commissioning is another attempt to engage clinicians in shaping specialist and community services to obtain better quality care for their patients, using budget management as the lever for change. In that sense its pedigree includes fundholding,[29] but the differences between PBC and the standard forms of fundholding are significant. First, the budget management is within a type 1 market where prices are fixed centrally through a national tariff to prevent price competition, and second, the range of services open to change is broader, and could include social care as well as medical and nursing services. Primary care itself is, therefore, subject to commissioning, requiring GPs to consider their own need and capacity to change the ways in which they work. This reflexivity is apparent in the features of commissioning plans, which should be based upon:

- How practices will respond to the particular need of their population and their patients' experiences of using the NHS.
- The practice's particular contribution to achieving waiting time targets for specialist services.
- How practices will contribute to the redesign of services and the resources that could be released as a result.
- Identifying aspects of health and social care where a collective approach across practices would be beneficial.

The experience of fundholding was an unhappy one, but it generates some new knowledge about commissioning processes to add to that emerging from other countries and services, and it is possible to see the potential benefits and risks of the comprehensive, psychosocial approach to service development that PBC represents. Box 2.2 summarizes some management perspectives on how PBC might alter general practice, community services, and hospital care, if it works at all.[30]

Box 2.2 Potential effects of practice-based commissioning

Benefits

- Lower elective referral and admission rates
- Reduced emergency-related bed days
- Lower waiting times for non-emergency treatment
- Improved co-ordination of primary, intermediate, and community support services
- Improvements in financial risk management
- Increased collaboration between general practices
- Slower growth of prescribing costs
- More engagement of clinicians in commissioning

Risks

- Reduced patient satisfaction (because practitioners' time, energy, and commitment are diverted)
- Increased management and transaction costs
- Inequities of access (because large practices will be better equipped to undertake PBC)
- Little impact on hospital care (beyond improving accessibility by shortening waiting times)

The risks are substantial, and the authors of this summary[30] argue that they can only be offset by practices combining together, in effect re-creating the PCGs that PCTs replaced.

There are a number of other major problems with the theory and practice of PBC. A recent overview of factors facilitating effective commissioning by primary care noted nine desirable characteristics of local health services[31] (see Box 2.3).

Box 2.3 Factors facilitating effective practice-based commissioning

1. Stability in the organization of healthcare, especially the structure of commissioning bodies

2. Sufficient time to enable clinicians to become engaged, and strategies for commissioning to be developed and implemented

3. Policy that supports offering patients and commissioners a choice of providers

4. Policy that enables resources to be shifted between providers and services

5. Real local choice in the provision of specialist services

6. Primary care developed enough to provide additional services

7. Incentives that motivate practitioners to change

8. Effective management to support PBC

9. Regulations that minimize conflicts of interest arising from GPs' dual role as providers and commissioners.

Despite noting that PBC is more likely to change primary than secondary care, the authors of the review see the policy context as more favourable for general practice engagement in commissioning than it was under the fundholding arrangement. This optimism may reflect their academic detachment; those with hands-on roles in running general practices scanning this list might be less positive about the potential of PBC.

While primary care is promoted as the driver of integrated care through its commissioning function, the professionals best placed to oversee this task may be experiencing changes in their work environment that will undermine their ability to carry it out.[32] It is far from clear that the managerial expertise needed to control a local health economy, cope with 'market failures' and address poor performance actually exists in present-day general practice, despite the rapid development that has occurred and even if a cadre of GPs separates off from clinical practice to take on the managerial role. However, the very nature of soft bureaucracy means that there is not likely to be a single outcome to the process of clinician engagement with managerial demands. Instead we could have multiple outcomes (which may increase the variations in service quality rather than reduce them), and multiple opportunities to shape general practice, so we should explore alternative approaches to the managerial challenges to clinician autonomy.

Alternative approaches

The view that service efficiency follows clinical effectiveness applies at the micro-level of the practice as much as at the macro-level of the whole service. If we think about promoting clinical effectiveness at practice or locality level we have two mechanisms that look promising as ways of preserving the primacy of clinical experience. The first is an alternative model of management to that of operating adhocracy, the J-shaped organization, and the second is a method for making economic judgements that reflect clinical perspectives, programme budgeting, and marginal analysis.

The J-shaped organization (the ideal Japanese work unit) accepts that knowledge should be standardized, but relies on teamwork, flexibility, a 'flat hierarchy' (i.e. a democratic internal culture), an emphasis on innovation and co-operation around shared values. The 'soft bureaucracy' of industrialization can be matched with a 'soft systems' approach to managing change,[33] which involves:

- Producing a detailed picture of the current situation, which highlights problems that have high priority.
- Identify possible solutions to problems, taking into account who would carry out and who would benefit from change, and what resistance and local constraints might be present.
- Creating a conceptual model of change, showing who is affected and involved.
- Checking the feasibility of the conceptual model against the original detailed description.
- Planning and implementing change.

This 'soft systems' approach could fit within the community oriented primary care idea that we will meet in Chapter 8, but its important feature is the conscious need to develop and sustain a management culture within the practice that engages all clinicians, but also as many practice members as possible. General practices can operate in such a way, but not without difficulties. J-shaped organizations need to think (which is difficult as a collective task), avoid scapegoating individuals (projecting failure or fault into susceptible individuals), and focus on work-tasks while allowing time and space for discussion of defences and basic assumptions that may impair the work task's implementation.

One view of such an approach to management[34] suggests that essential attributes include clarity about the task of the organization, clarity about the authority structure and regular opportunities to participate and contribute. Those in authority in such a work group need to have a psychologically-informed approach to management, an awareness of risks to workers, openness to service users' experiences, and a strong sense of public accountability.

The principles that could be applied to the practice could also help with collaboration between practices, if this is the best route to make PBC work. Because centrifugal forces are increasing within the NHS, collaboration between different organizations, disciplines, and groups is emphasized, but difficult to achieve. Simple rules include:[35]

- ◆ The task of the collaborative group must be clear and feasible.
- ◆ This task must not conflict with the tasks of the home groups.
- ◆ It must be important enough for collaboration group members to invest commitment and time to it.
- ◆ Home groups must invest time, resources and authority in the collaborative group.
- ◆ Membership of the collaboration group must be related to its task.
- ◆ A new management system develops to implement the collaborative group's task.

These capabilities could permit a kind of total quality management, in which the focus is on improving the whole organization in terms of efficient care (as seen through the eyes of the patient), optimal team-working, employee commitment, stabilizing the infrastructure and concentrating on the quality of care.[36] While we have to acknowledge that attempts to promote this in general practice have suggested that long-term, intensive external support (of a kind unlikely to be forthcoming in the current policy climate) is needed, and that results are modest,[37] we should also accept that such approaches to development and innovation need to be sustained for long periods of time before their outcomes can be assessed.

Programme budgeting and marginal analysis

Programme budgeting and marginal analysis is the kind of task that a collaborative group of practices could carry out. It is an approach to changing services that can accommodate clinical and managerial perspectives, together with wider professional, patient, and public opinion, in a single decision-making process.[38] An advisory panel needs to be constructed to reflect local stakeholder interests; we shall return to the possible composition of this panel in Chapter 7. Two economic concepts are used, opportunity costs (the costs of opportunities foregone) and marginal cost (the benefit gained or lost from have one extra unit more or less). This approach first examines current spending then considers the benefits and costs of changes by asking five questions, as shown in Box 2.4.

Box 2.4 Five questions about resource use

1. What are the total resources available?
2. Which services are being paid for currently?
3. What services are candidates for receiving more or new resources, and what are the costs and benefits of growth in these services?
4. Can any existing services be provided more efficiently, to release resources?
5. Can any services be reduced to release resources for growth areas that might offer greater benefit?

Programme budgeting and marginal analysis insert economic evaluation into a managerial structure such as that described above for PBC, creating a defensible mechanism for practitioners and managers to prioritize between national guidance or requirements and local needs. It is too slow and complex a process for the 'turn around' teams of accountants and managers struggling with massively overspent PCTs, but combined with the methods of public involvement discussed in Chapter 7 it could provide a framework for GP thinking in the next phase of industrialization. Before we can get to that discussion, however, we need to think about where GPs would fit in a redesigned system of primary care, by exploring another facet of industrialization, 'forward integration'.

References

1. Wainwright D. Disenchantment, ambivalence and the precautionary principle: the becalming of British health policy. *Int J Health Serv* 1998; **28**(3): 407–26.

2. Flynn R. 'Soft bureaucracy', governmentality and clinical governance: theoretical approaches to emergent policy. In *Governing medicine: theory and practice*. Gray A, Harrison S (eds). Maidenhead: Open University Press, 2004, pp. 11–26.

3. Courpasson D. Managerial strategies of domination: power in soft bureaucracies. *Organ Stud* 2000; **21**(1): 141–61.

4. Quoted in: Kmietowicz Z. One year to save the NHS: what would you do? *BMJ* 2007; **334**: 181.

5. Lucas K, Bickler G. Altogether now? Professional differences in the priorities of primary care groups. *J Public Health Med* 2000; **22**(2): 211–15.

6. Leese B. Impact on health authorities of the introduction of primary care groups and trusts. *Health Serv Manage Res* 2002; **15**: 40–5.

7. Craig N, McGregor S, Drummond N, Fischbacher M, Iliffe S. Factors affecting the shift towards a 'primary care led' NHS. *Br J Gen Pract* 2002; **52**(484): 895–900.

8. Thomas P, McDonnell J, McCulloch J, While A, Bosanquet N, Ferlie E. Increasing capacity for innovation in bureaucratic primary care organisations: a whole system action research project. *Ann Fam Med* 2005; **3**(4): 312–17.

9. Marshall M, Mannion R, Nelson E, Davies H. Managing change in the culture of general practice: qualitative case studies in primary care trusts. *BMJ* 2003; **327**: 599–602.

10. McCaffrey T. The pain of managing: the dynamics of the purchaser/provider split. in Foster A, Roberts Z, *Managing Mental Health in the Community*.

11. Thorne M. Colonising the new world of NHS management; the shifting power of professionals. *Health Serv Manage Res* 2002; **15**: 14–26.

12. Marshall M, Sheaff R, Rogers A, Campbell S, Halliwell S, Pickard S, Sibbald B, Roland M. A qualitative study fo the cultural changes in primary care organisations needed to implement clinical governance. *Br J Gen Pract* 2002: **52**: 641–5.

13. Checkland K, Harrison S, Marshall M. Is the metaphor of 'barriers to change' useful in understanding implementation? Evidence from general medical practice. *J Health Serv Res Policy* 2007; **12**(2): 95–100.

14. Rhydderch M, Elwyn G, Marshall M, Grol R. Organisational change theory and the use of indicators in general practice. *Qual Saf Health Care* 2004; **13**: 213–17.

15. Weick KE, Quinn RE. Organisational change and development. *Annu Rev Psychol* 1999; **50**: 361–86.

16. Van de Ven AH, Poole M. Explaining development and change in organisations. *Acad Manage Rev* 1995; 510–40.

17. McKee M, Sheldon T. Measuring performance in the NHS. *BMJ* 1998; **316**: 322.

18. Eddy D. Performance measurement: problems and solutions. *Health Affairs* 1998; **17**: 7–25.

19. Sheaff R, Rogers A, Pickard S, Marshall M, Campbell S, Sibbald B, Halliwell S, Roland M. A subtle governance: 'soft' medical leadership in English Primary Care. *Sociol Health Illness* 2003; **25**(5): 408–28.

20. Sennett R. *The corrosion of character*. London: Norton, 1998, p. 47.

21. Piore MJ, Sabel CF. *The second industrial divide: possibilities for prosperity*. New York: Basic Books, 1984, p. 17.

22. Harrison B. *Lean and mean*. New York: Basic Books, 1994, p. 47.

23. Stokes J. Institutional chaos and personal stress. In *The unconscious at work: individual and organisational stress in the human services*. Obholzer A, Roberts VZ (eds). London: Routledge, 1994, pp. 123–5.

24. Lam A. Tacit knowledge, organisational learning and societal institutions: an integrated framework. *Organ Stud* 2000; **21**: 487–513.

25. Smith J. *Report of the Chairman; Medical Defence Union Report, Accounts 2000*. London: MDU, 2001, p. 1.

26. Checkland K. Management in general practice: the challenge of the new General Medical Services contract. *Br J Gen Pract* 2004; **54**: 734–9.

27. Checkland K. Management in General Practice: the challenge of the new General Medical Services contract. *Br J Gen Pract* 2004; **54**(507): 734–9.

28. Midgley G. Systemic intervention for Public Health. *Am J Public Health* 2006; **96**(3); 466–72.

29. Walker N, Lorimer R. Practice based commissioning: technical briefing. *Commissioning News* No. 2 February 2007. http://www.commissioningnews.com/.

30. Greener I, Mannion R. Does practice based commissioning avoid the problems of fundholding? *BMJ* 2006; **333**: 1168–70.

31. Smith J, Dixon J, Mays N, *et al.* Practice based commissioning: applying the research evidence *BMJ* 2005; **331**: 1397–9.

32. Frusher T. Managing change: general practice and the transformation of primary care *Health Policy Rev* 2006; **3**: 44–58.

33. Checkland P, Scholes J. *Soft systems: methodology in action.* Chichester: John Wiley & Sons, 1990.

34. Obholzer A. Managing social anxieties in public sector organisations. In *The unconscious at work: individual and organisational stress in the human services.* Obholzer A, Roberts VZ (eds). London: Routledge, 1994, pp. 175–6.

35. Roberts VZ. Conflict and collaboration: managing intergroup relations. In *The unconscious at work: individual and organisational stress in the human services.* Obholzer A, Roberts VZ (eds). London: Routledge, 1994, p. 195.

36. Kenagy J, Berwick D, Shore M. Service quality in health care. *JAMA* 1999; **281**: 661–5.

37. Grol R. Improving the quality of medical care. *JAMA* 2007; **286**(20): 2578–85.

38. Ruta D, Mitton C, Bate A, Donaldson C. Programme budgeting and marginal analysis: bridging the gap between doctors and managers. *BMJ* 2005; **330**: 1501–3.

Chapter 3

Forward integration

Under a banner headline 'get competitive or go under' Doctor Newspaper reported RCGP Chairman Professor Mayur Lakhani as saying: 'The future will be competition on quality, not price–the laissez faire practice will be toast. The practice that succeeds is one that is patient-centred, focused on quality and has a learning culture.'
Doctor *(8 May 2007)*

British general practice faces three problems that are proving difficult to solve. The first is the growing volume and complexity of demands for medical care by citizens, driven by the forces discussed in Chapter 7. The second is the ageing of the workforce, with different career patterns built around part-time working and job mobility, and with pockets of recruitment difficulties emerging in both medicine and nursing.[1] The third is the failure of general practice to maintain its gatekeeper function for specialist services. This chapter will explore the third problem, considering its causes, reviewing solutions to it that have largely failed, and analysing three aspect of industrialization that may solve it and that are now well underway: skill mix changes, substitution of doctors by nurses, and the specialization of general practitioners (GPs) and practice or community nurses. These three approaches to changing work patterns are all part of the process of 'forward integration', and raise important questions about the ways in which team working will evolve.

Within an industrialized health service the purpose of 'forward integration' is to reposition all available resources so that they can be used to maximum technical efficiency (desired quality at lowest cost) as well as allocative efficiency (optimal mix for demand). 'Forward integration' of general practice within the health service seeks to make a whole and coherent production process out of disparate components, and requires changes in who does what, where; and in how they are organized, managed and, if necessary, paid.

The failure of gatekeeping

The failure of gatekeeping seems to be a failure that dare not speak its name, and discussions of specialization in general practice such as that of Nocon and Leese, published in the *British Journal of General Practice* in 2004,[2] are so detailed in their dissection of 'general practice with a special interest' (GPwSIs) that the reasons for its emergence as a policy concern are almost obscured. Yet the accounts of how GPwSIs can do some of the work of specialists, and the insistence that such endeavours are supplementing specialist care, not substituting for it, are indicators of high levels of inappropriate referrals and poor responses to management of long-term conditions in the community. At least a quarter of GP referrals to hospital chest clinics could be dealt with in general practice[3] (if it were more skilled and better organized), and 40–80% of ENT referrals may be similar.[2]

Let us look at another clinical example, the diagnosis and management of heart failure, a common clinical problem with a high morbidity and mortality, which can be successfully palliated with medication. The diagnosis cannot be made by clinical signs alone, requiring an echocardiogram. Management of heart failure in general practice is poor across Europe, and echocardiography is underutilized.[4] GPs attribute their overall poor performance to limited access to the crucial diagnostic test, lack of time, lack of expertise and anxieties about initiating treatment with angiotensin-converting inhibitors inhibitors.[5] The question is, why does a discipline that has a great deal of discretion in the way it works and organizes its time, and the freedom to invest its resources (money, time, and staff) as it chooses, not remedy this situation? Investment in the technology may be not something that individual practices would consider, but the aggregates of practices that made up multifunds in the first phase of industrialization and the locality commissioning structures that emerged then and are reviving now would be capable of such investments. The educational steps needed to know more, feel more comfortable with the diagnostic difficulties and the treatments available, and organize systematic care of this very needy patient group were all reinforced by the National Service Framework for Heart Disease. We shall see in Chapter 4 how variable responses to National Service Frameworks were.

The joint guidance from the department of Health and the Royal College of GPs lists 11 domains where there are 'access problems' to specialist care or where national priorities required greater medical input.[6] They are shown in Box 3.1

Box 3.1

- Cardiology
- Care of older people
- Palliative care and cancer
- Mental health, including substance misuse
- Dermatology
- Musculoskeletal medicine
- Women and children's health, and sexual health
- ENT medicine
- Services for those who find services hard to access—asylum seekers and travellers
- Diagnostic processes—endoscopies, cystoscopies, and echocardiograms
- Surgical procedures, such as vasectomy

Most of medicine is inside the box, only respiratory diseases, endocrine disorders, and neurology being domains that are not apparent in the list, and even some of them may fit within 'care of older people'. What the list says is that large parts of medical practice currently carried out by hospital specialists are within the competence of GPs interested enough to acquire a little extra knowledge and some extra skills. That interest exists within general practice. One estimate (published in 2002) suggested that there were about 4000 GPs already working as if they were GPwSIs, of whom only 19% had a contract with a primary care trust, health authority, or community trust. Most were working as hospital practitioners or clinical assistants, but a third had no contractual commitment to specialize, they just did it.[7] The question is, why are there not more GPwSIs already? If there are serious access issues to specialist care in some disciplines or areas, and the skills are within the range of GPs (4000 have already achieved it, to some extent), what has held back the development of specialization? We all know from experience about the frustration that patients express at having to wait a long time for, say, an ENT appointment is conveyed to their GP. We might add our own frustration, when we realize what is done in the ENT clinic is in part within the capabilities of general practice. What is hindering the rapid uptake of new knowledge and new roles?

It is not difficult to see how this has come about. It may not be possible for generalists to expand their practical knowledge across the range of medical problems that they encounter, as fast as the science itself evolves. Even if the pace of professional development could, in theory, keep up it would require the re-routing of time, energy, and money (for equipment) on a scale that is unlikely in a discipline organized in a way that favours conservative investment decisions. Some specialization occurs, of course, as professional enthusiasm drives individual GPs and whole practices to adopt new ways of working and new techniques for engaging with their clinical task, but it has not matched the scale of change in medical knowledge and technology. Our conservatism in making investment decisions results in a relative underskilling compared with specialists, who may collude with this underskilling (while also regretting it) because it keeps their expert identity secure and perhaps also their private practice plump.

A different funding system, and a less securely subordinate relationship to specialists, might have produced a different outcome, as in Germany, where the well-equipped practice will have direct access to diagnostic resources (e.g. ultrasound) and treatment options (e.g. physiotherapy) on a scale only imaginable in Britain.

Failed responses

Two responses to the growing demand for attention in general practice and the fragility of the gatekeeper function were tried, one before industrialization gained energy and one in its early phase. The first was to reduce general practice list sizes so that more time could be given to individual patients, particularly those with more complex problems. The second was to move specialists into general practice, in the kind of outreach arrangements that fundholding embraced.

Reducing list sizes was an ambition in general practice just before the industrialization process became overt, in the early 1990s. Many GPs seemed to believe that a reduction of list sizes towards 1700 patients per doctor was conducive to both better treatment for patients and better working conditions for doctors, the assumption being that patient demand shaped clinical activity and that GPs had little control over their work. Duncan Keeley, a London GP writing in the *British Medical Journal*[8] soon after the unilateral imposition of the first industrializing contract on general practice, quoted Professor Butler of the Health Services Research Unit at the University of Kent at Canterbury as saying: 'the argument that a continuing reduction in list sizes is a necessary precondition for an extension of a general practitioner's responsibilities is difficult to dispute'.

The government of the day did dispute it, stating in the Green Paper *Primary healthcare: an agenda for discussion* that: 'there is ... little evidence of a direct link between list size and the quality of care, and consequently there is little to indicate what might be the optimum list size'. Professor Butler and his colleague Michael Calnan published studies that tended to support the government's view, providing evidence that time released by list size reduction would be used to increase consultation rates (not lengths) and to reduce the length of the working week.[9] The demand-led model that GPs used to argue their case for improving the quality of care by reducing list sizes provided only a partial explanation for variations in time allocation in general practice.[10] In other words GPs had more control over their working time than they seemed to believe, or were prepared to speak about.

Duncan Keeley was prescient about the changes coming in general practice.[8]

> We are seeing the possibility of a major redefinition of the role of the general practitioner principal. The emphasis would be less on 'personal primary and continuing care of individuals and families and more on organizing the work of a team of (hierarchically inferior) health workers, deciding how the money for the healthcare of our patients should be spent, and keeping that expenditure within limits.'

Personal care, which has been something of a touchstone for general practice, was already fading away in group practices when he wrote. George Freeman, then an academic GP in Southampton, demonstrated in a study of four group practices that personal continuity of care was fairly low, especially for younger and healthier patients registered with practices with combined lists.[11] A decade later a large survey covering 53 general practices in four regions of the UK suggested that list sizes over 6500 were associated with marked reductions in personal continuity.[12] The prospect of improving the quality of care in general practice through list size reduction disappeared in the early phase of industrialization, and personal care—although still central to the ideology of general practice—is peripheral to its actual development.

Hospital outreach by specialists became popular as a potential solution to the skill shortage in general practice, particularly during the fundholding period. The logic seemed to be that moving specialists nearer to the 'coal face' (as if they did not work at one already) would function as a kind of triage for further investigation and educate the GPs at the same time. There is some evidence that the processes of care (waiting times, patient satisfaction, convenience to patients, follow-up attendances) were better in outreach clinics than in outpatient clinics. However, waiting lists were usually not reduced by organizing outreach clinics, costs (in travelling time) for specialists increased and a two-tier service threatened.[13] A later review of the evidence suggested that specialist outreach did not reduce outpatient demand, but did improve access in remote areas, while the quality of care could deteriorate if GPs undertook more minor surgery.[14] It is hardly surprising that outreach by mainstream specialists has dwindled, to be replaced by nurse practitioner outreach for specific conditions, such as heart failure and respiratory diseases, which we will return to later in this chapter.

There remains an increasingly urgent need to re-establish a gatekeeper function, while at the same time responding to the understandings and expectations of an increasingly knowledgeable, articulate and assertive population. As the composition and strengths of local primary care workforces vary so much, there is no logical reason to think that any one approach will fit all. Inevitably commissioners of primary care will need to try different models for size and fit in their workforce, and this is exactly what the national health service (NHS) is attempting through changing skill mix, attempting the substitution of GPs by nurses and the supplementation of specialist care by generalists. Even if the evidence base for each is thin, these approaches seem worth considering because of their plausibility and intellectual coherence, their concordance with current policy objectives and their potential to meet several different needs simultaneously.

Changing the skill mix

Changing the composition of a workforce by altering the proportions of different skills has been found to be effective, especially in nursing,[15] but it is difficult to know if it is cost-effective because the economic consequences of releasing one professional's time are complex and not always well understood. For example, a reduction in the proportion of one professional group—say, district nurses—and their replacement by cheaper healthcare assistants may seem 'economic', but savings may be offset by the need to use incentives to attract district nurses into such a re-configured team. The prospect of managing a small team of assistants may seem more attractive than carrying a large case load of hands-on work, but this satisfaction could be reduced if the assistants are poorly trained or inexperienced, if they stay only a short time in the job (because of its difficulties, the low pay and the hours), or if the case load is too large and the team is spread too thinly. The more expensive option—having an experienced, high-grade nurse manage a case load directly—might be the more stable arrangement that provides higher quality care and produces the most job satisfaction. GPs will have encountered this problem many times, with locums who see the requisite number of patients but create more work for the practice through referrals that subsequently seem unnecessary, or through re-visits by patients who did not get their usual care. A GP Registrar or an FY2 (Foundation Year 2) doctor may seem to be an asset, in terms of helping reduce the workload, but that all depends on their clinical and interpersonal skills, and the degree of supervision they need.

The size and mix of the primary care workforce in any locality are determined by factors that are 'historical and irrational at best'.[16] As workforce planning rises up the agenda for primary care organizations (including large practices) in response to rising demand, local organizations become more complex, which complicates planning. A single-handed GP can make decisions about practice management and organization without consulting anyone, and can therefore make rapid changes. A small team will have a short decision-making cycle, but this will lengthen as the team size increases, and become more complex if the range of disciplines increases. A large medical centre with GPs as the 'owning' co-operative, plus practice nurses, psychologists or counsellors, management and administration staff as employees, and other doctors, health visitors, district nurses, and community psychiatric nurses in attached or liaison roles, is likely to have a long decision-making cycle and consultation processes that can easily go wrong.

The problem with the skill mix concept is that it has a limited evidence base. There is a lack of clarity about the strategic objectives of changing skill mix, and it is much harder to see the real differences between disciplines (for example, doctors and nurses) than the professions like to think.[17] The strongest evidence for changing the skill mix is the growth in the numbers of nurse practitioners and physicians assistants in the USA. These two disciplines make up one-sixth of the US healthcare workforce and offer a range of services equivalent to 90% of a family physician's role. Their education time is approximately half that of physicians and their entry into the workforce is less restrictive. Fifty per cent of physician assistants and

85% of nurse practitioners work in primary care services, compared with only 30% of doctors.[18]

Substitution

There are different estimates of the amount of work done by GPs that could be done by nurses. One study found that 39% of GP consultations contained at least one task that could be done by a nurse, and 17% were entirely suitable for a nurse,[1] although with significant misgivings in both disciplines.[19] Another estimate suggested that between 30% and 70% of tasks undertaken by GPs could be carried out by nurses.[17]

Substitution of nurses for doctors has the potential to reduce both GP workload and costs, but not in all settings. The workload of the GP may remain unchanged because nurses are deployed to meet previously unmet need or because nurses generate demand for services where previously there was none. Savings will depend on the magnitude of salary differences between nurses and doctors—which may change according to supply and demand—and may also be offset by the lower productivity of nurses.[20] There is, however, only fragmented evidence to support such an approach to professional substitution, which is not necessarily cost-effective, or necessarily a source of better care, or even (for nurses) an automatic gain in professionalism.[21] The substitution of nurse's labour for doctor's labour may not be real, despite the intention, and may change into supplementation of medical care by a different, perhaps more advanced, form of practice nursing.[22] Some technologies may have the potential to facilitate substitution of one practitioner by another. For example, telephone consultation (by nurses) appears to reduce the number of surgery contacts and out-of-hours visits by GPs, but its effects on wider service use, safety, cost, and patient satisfaction need further study.[23]

Outside the clinical domain, in the management of services, GPs and primary care nurses may well be interchangeable, but even then the differences in professional cultures show through, with nurses being oriented more towards fostering teamwork and GPs focusing on leadership and delegation.[24] Although the boundaries of substitution are not known, there are strong arguments for adequate training, assessment and quality control systems if advanced roles for primary care nurses are to be widely introduced,[25] all of which are likely to reduced productivity and increase costs. The logic of substitution is, nevertheless, very attractive because it offers the possibility that some (undesired) work can be taken away from GPs, allowing more time for more appropriate or interesting work. Anxious parents with hot and miserable children, for example, can be seen, reassured and treated by a nurse practitioner trained in the management of minor illness, while the GP gets on with work that demands more medical expertise. In all this we need to remember the exemplary story of the Langwith village surgery, first mentioned in the introduction. It was the failure of a nurse-led service established by the Primary Care Trust to provide adequate care, together with the reluctance of local GPs to get involved, that led to the involvement of the private company United Health Europe, and the subsequent mobilization of professional and public opinion around an NHS solution.[26]

General practitioners with a special interest

GPwSIs may need to be very political creatures. Their success is likely to depend on gaining trust and credibility[27] and negotiating their way into local services,[28] but also with an eye to national priorities for health service development which will favour GPwSI deployment.[29] GPwSIs will need to tread carefully. Their special interest groups make it clear that they should not attempt to substitute for real specialists,[30] as such a challenge would probably provoke a response from hospital doctors that would jeopardize the further development of specialist roles for generalists.[2] Although there is little evidence that GPwSIs can improve quality of care or mediate in primary/secondary care boundary setting, they are nevertheless being promoted to reduce both waiting times and the use of secondary services.[31] The optimism about GPwSIs is grounded in their availability (in some places) to attempt to achieve policy targets such as waiting time reductions, their ability to improve the accessibility of specialist services,[32] and their potential as recruiting agents for general practice.

GPwSIs may enhance job satisfaction in general practice, and so improve recruitment and retention in the discipline, and could even become part of an increasingly flexible career structure that sees GPs and specialists have much more interchangeable career paths.[33] The integration of specialism and generalism need not be restricted to clinical domains, public health could also benefit from having GPwSIs.[34] However, the risks that GPwSIs run are also numerous. Not only might they deskill their colleagues without special interests, but they may also appear more frequently in areas of lowest need,[33] so adding to the irrationality of the primary care workforce rather than subtracting from it. They may turn out to be more expensive, as in one study of dermatology GPwSIs,[35] and require increasing amounts of resources in training, support systems, and the paraphernalia of clinical governance.[27] Finally, and crushingly, they may increase the overall workload by treating previously undertreated or even untreated conditions[33] and fail to reduce demands for specialist care.[2]

Case management of long-term conditions

If the benefits of encouraging GPs to become quasi-specialists are uncertain, could the NHS use nurses to do something similar? Nurses are certainly seen as a group that might take 'naturally' to case management approaches that focus clinical effort on managing complex people with complex problems. The management of long-term conditions and chronic diseases is arguably the main challenge for primary care, worldwide.[36] Individuals with long-term conditions consume a large proportion of health and social care resources, including 60% of hospital bed days in British hospitals,[37] and 78% of all healthcare spending in the USA. It is estimated 17.5 million adults in the UK are living with a chronic disease and that the incidence of chronic diseases and disabilities (long-term conditions) among those aged over 65 will double by 2030.[37,38]

Given the distribution of disease and disability a focus on later life is appropriate. In the early phase of industrialization this focus was managed badly, by pushing policy far ahead of evidence. As a result clinical practitioners in Britain may be wary of approaching systematic approaches to a whole population group such as those with chronic conditions, given the failure of population screening for untreated morbidity in older people. Not only did the '75 and over checks' introduced in 1990 have little discernible impact on the health of older people,[39] but the recent Medical Research Council trial of screening older people showed no benefits from such screening.[40] Neither GPs nor specialists in care of older people performed well in the Medical Research Council trial, suggesting that medical management of problems revealed by screening is essentially ineffectual. However, there is some evidence from studies in the USA that *targeted* needs assessment of older people followed by active management may improve both survival and functional ability.[41]

In North America comprehensive geriatric assessment with subsequent systematic management reduces hospital admission rates, and models of chronic disease management have evolved to exploit this impact and contain care costs for an ageing population. Whole systems approaches in the USA, using case management methods,[42,43] have been championed as a means of ensuring continuity of care, improving patient outcomes and achieving efficient management of resources.[44] The core elements of any case management activity are: identification of individuals likely to benefit from case management, assessment of the individual's problems and need for services, care planning of activities and services to address the agreed needs, referral to and co-ordination of services and agencies to implement a care plan, and regular review, monitoring, and consequent adaptation of the care plan.

The NHS is being encouraged to embark on a chronic disease management programme built around fostering self-management, enhancing disease management in primary care, and introducing case management for individuals with complex problems who make high use of hospital services.[37] The Royal Colleges of Physicians and of GPs and the NHS Alliance have endorsed this programme and have made proposals for joint clinical directorates and clinical governance, across the specialist–generalist divide.[44]

In the UK nurses are seen as the professional discipline with the abilities to carry out and co-ordinate chronic disease management, and chronic disease management is seen as one of the three core roles of primary care nurses. This is logical, as nurses have always been involved with people with chronic diseases through health promotion, patient teaching, direct nursing care, and the application of medical treatments. The current expectation that nurses will take greater responsibilities for the day to day care for people with chronic diseases, long-term disabilities, and complex needs is only an extension of a familiar role. This expectation is expressed in England by the drive to appoint 3000 'community matrons' to support people with complex long-term conditions using case management techniques, by 2007.[38] Their task will be to identify need, achieve continuity of care, promote coherence of services and review the quality of the care provided.[45]

Is this new approach to healthcare a decisive breakthrough in person-centred service provision, and are new case management roles for nurses in the community likely to be welcomed, effective and worthwhile? While there are good reasons for exploring the potential for nurse-led case management, we should be cautious about the political emphasis given to chronic disease management and expectations of nurse-led case management within it. Chronic disease management remains problematic as a model of care, with evidence from the USA of limited effectiveness, reliance on traditional forms of patient education, poor linkages to primary care and dependence on referrals rather than active case-finding approaches.[46] In the UK primary care organizations should be able to overcome some of the negative features of American experience, simply because we still have an integrated and resourced system of primary care, with a relatively influential discipline of public health. But we may not be able to overcome them all, for a number of reasons.

First, there is some doubt about whether chronic disease management is wanted by all patients. Patient priorities may differ from those NHS managers and clinicians, and older people who may feel that their independence and autonomy are threatened by an intrusive care system.[47] Nurses involved in public health drives such as influenza immunization, or disease management tasks such as diabetes and chronic obstructive pulmonary disease care, will have experienced the scale and persistence of resistance in people with long-term problems.

Secondly, there is the problem of how to identify those who are likely to need high levels of care, for there is no linear and unambiguous link between the presence of a condition that can be labelled chronic and the need for health or social care.[48] Patients with multiple emergency admissions ('frequent fliers') are often identified as a high-risk group for subsequent admission and substantial claims are made for interventions—such as case management—designed to avoid such admissions. However, simply monitoring admission rates cannot assess the effectiveness of case management, as admission rates fall without any intervention.[49] Promotion of case management on the basis of before and after comparisons of admission rates is, therefore, reliant on potentially flawed evidence.

Thirdly, case management as a technique is not a single or simple entity, there being several different types that require different types of work organization, demand different skills, and respond to different needs. For example, there are traditional forms of case management based on discipline or clinical speciality, such as district nursing; social services led care management, involving nurses; specialist nurses supporting people with particular diseases or conditions, such as heart failure or COPD nurses operating out of hospital departments or practice nurses focusing on care of patients with diabetes or asthma; and specialist nurses for the case management of people with multiple conditions. They are all carrying out different levels of case management work, but they are not necessarily interchangeable.

Finally, nurses may not be the best professionals to carry out chronic disease management as currently understood, despite the historic role of the discipline and the attractive logic of extending nursing roles. Studies that have compared nurse-led case management with case management led by other disciplines provide mixed evidence as to whether nurses achieve equivalent or better outcomes. Invariably, the studies lack detail about the nursing contribution, their exact roles, activities, and the expertise used.[50,51] There is, therefore, an urgent need to study the actual content of case management activities, and to mount the comparative studies that will reveal the optimal configuration of competencies for chronic disease management.

The current policy emphasis on chronic disease management will require extensive changes in service provision, significant re-training of staff, and widespread re-negotiation of relationships between disciplines and agencies. The opportunities for innovation are huge, and the potential for rigorous evaluation of new approaches to care is great, so both primary care practitioners and researchers will be busy as the 'community matrons' get to work. The risks are equally great, for health service policy could be decided prematurely, so that particular models of chronic disease management are promoted on the basis of superficial assessment, political attractiveness, or organizational expediency. We are at risk of repeating the errors of the '75 and over checks' policy, which was introduced in 1990 against the advice of the profession and took 14 years to undo. General practice as a discipline has one big advantage that may prevent another policy failure; its experience of team working.

Team working

If one of the persistent problems of general practice has been its conservative approach to investment, one of its strengths has been its interest in multidisciplinary working, once financial incentives were in place to sustain it. We might envy our German peers with their ultrasound machines in their offices, but we can be proud of the wide range of co-workers that we have and that European generalists (as a whole) lack. Collaboration and team work have long been advocated[52,53] as a means of providing effective primary healthcare. However, there is an equally long history of critically assessing the reality behind the rhetoric of teamwork in primary healthcare,[54,55] Many commentators have pointed to employment status differences, professional cultural differences, geographical separation, and membership of multiple teams as real barriers to team working.[56–58]

The most obvious example of team development in general practice is the shift in workload from GPs to practice nurses and nurse practitioners.[59] The requirements of the 1990 GP contract, together with the administration of fundholding, led to the phenomenal growth in the direct employment of administrative staff and nurses in general practice.[60] The emergence of the general practice as a powerful unit in purchasing and/or commissioning health services influenced closer working arrangements between community nurses and practices, including experiments with integrated nursing teams.[61,62] Around the same time the NHS and Community Care Act 1990,[63] legislated for collaboration in planning and delivering individuals' care as well as service planning. This was later reinforced by the establishment of Primary Care Groups [64] in 1997, based on collaboration between different professional groups in the planning, provision and monitoring of healthcare services for small populations.

In the first phase of industrialization the impetus to team-working was part pragmatic (with GPs delegating a widening workload) and part idealistic. There appeared at the time to be little direct evidence of benefits to patients from greater team-working in primary care,[65] but from other domains there was evidence of more efficient health-care delivery and increased staff motivation,[66] and this was good enough to promote innovative ways of working. An intuitive list of the benefits of collaborative working included beliefs that:

- Care given by a group is greater than that given by one.
- Rare skills and knowledge are used more appropriately in teams.
- Duplication and gaps in care giving and other activities are avoided by team-working.
- Peer influence and informal learning occur within teams and raise standards of care.
- Team members have greater job satisfaction and are better able to cope with the stresses of working in primary care.
- Teams contain the potential for developing more creative and lateral solutions to problems.

The possibilities that arose from collaborative working between disciplines were attractive given the anxieties that were emerging about the sustainability of health service delivery in its usual forms. A joint statement on team-working in primary care published in 2000 by the Royal Pharmaceutical Society of Great Britain and the British Medical Association pointed out that the number of professionals (especially doctors) was unlikely to be sufficient to meet expectations for timely provision of high quality care if services continued to be organized in traditional ways.[67] In other words, team-working was not just intrinsically desirable, but essential to avoid a crisis in primary care. However, the report also points out that, despite the catalytic role of some professionals in different disciplines in promoting team-work, the first major obstacle to collaboration was professionalism itself. The second was the lack of a shared information technology that would allow the emergence of a common electronic patient record.

The potential for a coherent, efficient, and collaborative system of patient care existed, but the historically determined relationships between disciplines combined with the plurality of incompatible IT systems meant that this potential could not easily be realized.

If the report from the Royal Pharmaceutical Society of Great Britain and the British Medical Association is correct, overcoming the barriers to collaborative working is one of the main challenges for primary care, and so for general practice. Seen from the perspective of industrialization, it is a core component of 'forward integration'. There seem to be three important aspects to team-working that need to be addressed; organizational forms and the distribution of managerial power between disciplines, location and team size, and the nature and depth of the desired collaboration.

Organization, management, and power

The Royal College of General Practitioners[68] distinguishes between a core primary care team of GPs and employees of the practice and the wider multiprofessional network outside the direct control of the GPs. Those who are collaborators in the provision of health and social care for some or all of the practice population—community nurses and health visitors, midwives, psychologists, counsellors—but managed and paid by other organizations are likely to have different approaches to team-working than the core group, if only because their management can require them to work in ways that the GPs do not determine. There is also a second distinction to be made between the members of the core team who are partners in the financial business of the practice, and those who are directly employed by the practice. In an industrializing health service where efficiency is paramount, those inside the economic co-operative lose income if team-working does not deliver gains in efficiency and quality of care, while those who are employed by the co-operative continue to earn the same salaries. Similarly, salaried employees may increase the efficiency and quality of care, within a new division of labour between disciplines, and see the financial benefits go to the partners within the co-operative. We shall see how this occurred during the MMR controversy when health visitors came to experience themselves as agents of GPs driven by targets. These distinctions are one of the biggest potential sources of tension in the entity called a 'primary healthcare team', and are the subject of continuous debate within the industrialization process. GPs weigh up the merits of being salaried employees or dependent contractors, practices consider the kind of contract that they hold with primary care organizations, primary care trusts explore ways of divesting themselves of responsibility for managing community nursing and other disciplines and GPs think about employing physiotherapists or midwives.

Locality and team size

Physical proximity, social proximity, and positive motivation are prerequisites to collaboration and team working, as is (obviously) interaction between members.[69] Repeated studies from the 1960s onwards have shown that collaboration is closest between GPs and district nurses and health visitors when the nurses are physically based in the same building and are attached to no more than two general practices.[70] The ability to have an impromptu discussion in the corridor or the car park about a patient, or a decision that affects the team, must lubricate the processes of collaboration and add value to the ability to meet more formally and work through agendas, or at least so we think in general practice. Other disciplines may not agree. There is evidence from a study of collaboration between social workers and GPs[71] that co-location is seen by social workers as potentially isolating, and a challenge to social work practice, because the team working desired by GPs required social workers to adapt their behaviour and thinking to those of family medicine. The shift in thinking was from the 'holding' orientation of social work to the 'action orientation' of general practice;[72] the doctors wanted 'something to be done' while the social workers wanted to consider the options more carefully.

The size of the team's membership also appears to be an important factor, with three to six offered as the most effective group size for decision-making and communicating.[73] This desirable size, which matches the optimal size for practices trying to maintain continuity of care, has implications for the much larger teams now emerging in general practice.

Levels of collaboration

There are different ways to think about and describe the levels of collaborative work in primary care teams.[74] These range from complete isolation, where clinical information, referral or requests are passed between doctors, nurses, and social workers via administrative staff or relatives, so that the professionals never talk or meet, to full collaboration, where professionals' work is fully integrated across disciplines, at the other end of the scale. Looked at another way we can define three levels of team working:[75]

- The nominal team, characterized by isolated working by professionals.
- Convenient teams, in which tasks are delegated down a hierarchical structure.
- Committed teams, characterized by fully integrated working between disciplines.

All of these arrangements can be functional, both from the viewpoint of the professions concerned and from the perspective of those using services. In circumstances of high demand and relatively low resources streamlined working with limited communication is adopted for sake of efficiency. The most effective team-building work appears to take place when there is a clear practice-based project to be undertaken,[76] so practices facing increasing demands to standardize and improve the quality of care have developed convenience teams to tackle Quality Outcomes Framework targets and manage patient demand. The committed team may emerge around a shared desire to optimize palliative care, or the management of patients with mental health problems, or the care of older people. What can be achieved in terms of collaborative working is dependent upon demand and resources, mediated by the enthusiasm of professionals for joint working, but we always need to be conscious of the limits of our knowledge. If we take collaborative working between primary care and social services as an example, we should recognize that there is as yet little evidence that closer working results in higher quality care, cheaper services, or more satisfied patients.[77] This is not an argument against collaboration, but a reminder that all attempts at joint working, even within small groups where shared objectives are more likely to exist, are exploratory and experimental.

Conflict in teams

Paradoxically, while team work can contribute to high levels of job satisfaction it can also be a source of stress for individuals. Teamwork can expose role ambiguity and opposing values. It is, however, interpersonal conflict that can lead to the most intractable stress for individual members.[78] In primary care, the multiple professional groupings add particular dimensions for interpersonal conflict and it would be naive to underestimate this. So not only are there possibilities for conflict within one group—(for example, the partners in the practice)—but also between groups, such as the practice nurses, district nurses, and health visitors, who are all technically nurses working in the community.

The corporate image of a team, according to Sennett, is 'a group of people assembled to perform a specific, immediate task, rather than to dwell together as a village ... a worker has to bring to short-term tasks an instant ability to work well with a shifting cast of characters'.[79] The social skills needed must be portable (from team to team and project to project) and some detachment is required, so that the worker can stand back from established relationships and judge how they can be changed. This idea of a team fits to some extent with experience in group general practice. The specific and immediate tasks are not projects emerging in the market, but responses to the demands of a shifting cast of characters, the patient population. This population is shifting in all kinds of ways—in age, in knowledge and experience, in work, in relationships, and in domicile. However, the team may dwell together as a village, to some extent, although not literally. Working relationships may vary between close, extending outside work, to distant, with no extra-mural contact. Standing back from relationships with patients is problematic, as the knowledge acquired by both parties over a period of time can be important to the solution of problems—the succession of specific and immediate tasks. Part-time working, reduced hours (e.g. withdrawal from out-of-hours work) and group working all help to break up long-term relationships, contributing to the shifting cast of characters.

The US Secretary of Labor's Commission on achieving necessary skills, reporting in 1991, emphasized communication and facilitation in teams.[80] Teamwork may be presented as 'a culture of co-operation (promoted) through egalitarian symbols',[81] but may also function as a form of deep acting,[82] creating masks of co-operation that establish the friendliness of the worker rather than his/her genuine concern with the other person's problem. 'In a turnstile world of work, the masks of co-operativeness are among the only possessions that workers will carry with them from task to task.'[83] General practice is very much a turnstile world. Do we struggle to promote masks of co-operation in reception staff? Even the appearance of co-operativeness may be difficult to sustain, given the tendency of people to fit their own anxieties to their work, and use work to resolve personal problems, sometimes through self-imposed impossible tasks.[84]

Team-working practices are a continuum, from uni-professional teams at the novice end, through multidisciplinary teams, to interprofessional working at the expert end of professional development.[85] Interprofessional working implies a shared learning experience with, from, and about each other.[86] Progression along the continuum involves a reduction in professional autonomy and an increase in shared expertise.[87] Team tasks need to be clear, motivating, and consistent with group purpose,[88] intrinsically interesting with meaningful and inherent rewards,[89] and subject to shared concerns about quality, vision, outcomes, and evaluation.[90] Team leadership involves focusing efforts towards a common goal.[91] Models of shared, rotating or distributed leadership have merged in healthcare.[92] Leadership requires the maintenance of a balance between the task, the group, and the individual,[93] involving attention to team membership, integration, and management.[94] However, the provision of health services is characterized by high levels of uncertainty and complexity, creating challenges for establishing clear goals[95] (especially in general practice). Engel points out that, in healthcare, motivation needs to be essentially intrinsic and collaborating in teams offers only limited reward.[96]

One problem with modern teams is the repudiation of authority and the presentation of leaders as coaches or facilitators. This type of leadership shifts responsibility on to the workers' shoulders and makes everyone contingent on change, de-personalizing power.[97] This apparent neutrality is a form of betrayal, allowing those in control to focus on the present and act as they want without justification. This game of power without authority replaces the driven individual of the protestant work ethic with ironic man, who takes nothing and no one seriously because everyone is contingent. Such an individual is not quite real, and has no durable needs that others can meet; s/he cannot challenge power, and becomes self-destructive.[98] 'Irreversible change and multiple, fragmented activity may be comfortable for the regime's masters, ... but it may disorientate the regime's servants. And the new co-operative ethos of teamwork sets in place as masters those "facilitators" ... who dodge truthful engagement with their servants.'[99]

One issue that is avoided in the modern concept of teamwork is the importance of conflict. We are bound together more by conflict than by agreement, although we can reach agreement through conflict. Conflict requires harder work at communication, the rules of engagement bring people together, individuals and groups become better at listening and responding, and differences can be clarified even as agreement is reached.[100] Strong communities address differences, over time, making current ideas of teamwork sources of weak community feeling. The evolving expression of disagreement engages people more than the declaration of correct principles.[101]

Pragmatic solutions

The temptation for practitioners is to anticipate that we can, individually, recapture the generalist ability to carry out many different tasks and be a Jack or Jill of all trades. It is possible to describe the variety of work in general practice in terms of the palette of skills that generalists master and deploy, as in this account: 'Diverse diagnostic challenges such as reviewing the diabetic retina, inspecting the cervix, making sense of multiple non-specific symptoms, assessing the suicide risk in a depressed young man, and carrying out a developmental check on a newborn baby are just part of the normal working day for the medical generalist.'[102]

The problem with this inventory is that it may not actually fit with the 'normal working day' of many GPs, who have long since delegated the cervical smear test and the newborn baby check to practice nurses and midwives or health visitors respectively, while leaving retinal screening of patients with diabetes to ophthalmic opticians who have the necessary training and technology. It is difficult to see what advantage a GP has over a practice nurse in carrying out cervical cancer screening, or over a health visitor in carrying out child development assessments, and the performance of generalists in fundoscopy is poor enough to make it hazardous to leave this aspect of tertiary prevention to them. From this list only the diagnostic task—making sense of multiple symptoms—and the severity assessment (in depression) remain unchallenged within the generalist job description. These tasks, very much about interpreting situations and finding meanings, could be the only ones that we cannot delegate, and would therefore be the core business of general practice. We might add to the list of uncertainties the best way to prevent, identify, or manage diseases and disabilities in the community, returning once again to the arguments for integrating family medicine and public health in Tudor Hart's *New kind of doctor*.[103]

Perhaps the important point for us to remember is that we are not simply not specialists, but in some senses *antispecialists* (just as we are antimarket as long as we stay within the public domain). Anthony Giddens argues that the specialization that has made modern life in industrialized societies so rich also creates huge problems in interpreting knowledge, which in turn destabilize the understanding and confidence of many citizens. Specialization is a problem, as this quotation from *Modernity & self-identity* suggests:[104] '... expertise itself is increasingly more narrowly focused, and is liable to produce unintended and unforeseen outcomes which cannot be contained—save for the development of further expertise, thereby repeating the same problem.'

The rumour of a connection between the MMR vaccine and autism, when given the authority of an expert medical journal, was enough to reduce vaccine uptake to levels low enough to permit re-establishment of the diseases in some places, just as Giddens might predict. I will return to the MMR episode when discussing consumerism, in Chapter 7. To close the gap between what is possible to do in community settings given the current level of medical knowledge, and the actual performance of GPs and community nurses, we need to embrace the agenda of forward integration. There is a spectrum of professional activity based on the complexity of the tasks and the individual's ability to manage uncertainty. We will need to take a pragmatic approach to thinking about changing skill mix, based on strategic aims, perspectives, opinions, scope, likely costs and local views and experiences.[17]

Payment systems

Given that new forms of organization of community services in general, and of GPs' work in particular, are emerging, we may also have to consider different ways of funding our clinical, administrative and public health work. One argument in this chapter is that the franchise model of general practice, which had such advantages in the early period of the NHS by providing a localizing aspect to a nationalizing enterprise, lacks the mechanisms to support widespread and rapid changes in practice. The investment decisions that are typical of small-scale co-operatives working within a franchise structure to meet complex demands favour small-scale innovation, not system-wide modernization.

The puzzle that the NHS has now to work out is how to make investment decisions in primary care speedily enough for general practice to catch up with specialist medicine, without overburdening practitioners and losing their professional commitment, and without breaking the bank. One option might be to encourage salaried general practice, perhaps at locality level, to reduce the number of decision-makers in the field and give managers greater control over practitioners. Another—which has been adopted with the 2004 new General Medical Services contract -is to micro-manage consultations in selected clinical domains through a complex incentive system of targets. The policy problem for the NHS is that, when thinking of how to get the most appropriate package of skills within primary care, it needs to juggle productivity, professional enthusiasm, quality of care, and costs.

There is some evidence to suggest that the method of payment affects clinical behaviour. A systematic review of (rather meagre) evidence suggests that fee for service payments result in more primary care contacts, and greater use of diagnostic and curative services, but fewer hospital referrals and repeat prescriptions.[105] A Norwegian study of parallel contracts in general practice showed that family doctors with a fee for service contract have more consultations than those with a salaried contract, partly because they work longer hours and partly through working more efficiently. Salaried GPs preferred shorter working hours and less intensive work. The authors calculate that a change from a salaried to a fee for service contract would increase productivity by something between 2 and 40%.[106] An early comparison of PMS and General Medical Services practices in England came to a different conclusion, with no significant differences being found between the practice types in time worked, consultation lengths, prescribing, or referral rates.[107] Fee for service payment systems appear to offer more advantages for the health service (through increased productivity) but possibly less patient satisfaction.[108] There is little evidence to help decide whether target payment remuneration provides a mechanism for improving the quality of primary care.[109] One view on getting the right balance of contractual arrangements would be to assign the responsibility for contract-setting to local rather than national authorities, tailoring the incentives in the contract package according to local supply and demand.[110]

References

1. Jenkins-Clarke S, Carr Hill R. Changes, challenges and choices for the primary health care workforce: looking to the future. *J Adv Nurs* 2001; **34**(6): 842–9.

2. Nocon A, Leese B. The role of UK general practitioners with special clinical interests: implications for policy and service delivery. *Br J Gen Pract* 2004; **54**: 50–6.

3. Gilbert R, Franks G, Watkin S. The proportion of general practitioner referrals to a hospital respiratory medicine clinic suitable to be seen in a GPwSI respiratory clinic. *Prim Care Respir J* 2005; **14**(6): 314–19.

4. Khunti K, Hearnshaw H, Baker R, Grimshaw G. Heart failure in primary care: qualitative study of current management and perceived obstacles to evidence-based diagnosis and management by general practitioners. *Eur J Heart Fail* 2002; **4**(6): 771–7.

5. Fuat A, Hungin P, Murphy J. Barriers to accurate diagnosis and effective management of heart failure: qualitative study. *BMJ* 2003; **326**(7382): 196.

6. Department of Health, Royal College of General Practitioners. *Implementing a scheme for general practitioners with special interests*. London, 2003 http://www.doh.gov.uk/pricare/gp-specialinterests/gpwsiframework.pdf/.

7. Jones R, Bartholomew J. General practitioners with special clinical interests: a cross sectional survey. *Br J Gen Pract* 2002; **52**: 833–4.

8. Keeley D. Personal care or the Polyclinic? *BMJ* 1991; **302**: 1514–16.

9. Butler JR, Calnan MW. List sizes and the use of time ingeneral practice. *BMJ* 1987; **295**: 1383–6.

10. Calnan M, Butler J. The economy of time in general practice: an assessment of the influence of list size. *Soc Sci Med* 1988; **26**(4): 435–41.

11. Freeman G, Richards S. How much personal care in four group practices? *BMJ* 1990; **301**: 1028–30.

12. Guthrie B. Continuity in UK general practice: multilevel model of patient, doctor and practice factors associated with patients seeing their usual doctor. *Fam Pract* 2002; **19**(5): 496–9.

13. Bowling A, Stramer K, Dickson E, Windsor J, Bond M. Evaluation of specialists' outreach clinics in general practice in England: process and acceptability to patients, specialists and general practitioners. *J Epidemiol Community Health* 1997; **51**: 52–61.

14. Roland M, McDonald R, Sibbald B, Boyd A, Fotaki M, Gravelle H, Smith L. *Outpatient services and primary care. A scoping review of research into strategies for improving outpatient effectiveness and efficiency.* Report for the NHS Service delivery, Organisation R&D Programme, London, 2006.

15. Richardson J. Identifying, evaluating and implementing cost-effective skill mix. *Nurs Manage* 1999; **7**(5): 265–70.

16. Hurst K. Primary and community care workforce planning and development. *J Adv Nurs* 2006; **55**(6): 757–69.

17. Kernick D, Scott A. Economic approaches to doctor/nurse skill mix: problems, pitfalls and partial solutions. *Br J Gen Pract* 2002; **52**: 42–6.

18. Hooker RS. Physician assistants and nurse practitioners: the United States experience. *Med J Aust* 2006; **185**: 4–7.

19. Jennings-Clarke S, Carr-Hill R, Dixon P. Teams and seams: skill mix in primary care. *J Adv Nurs* 1998; **28**(5): 1120–6.

20. Laurent M, Reeves D, Hermens R, Braspenning J, Grol R, Sibbald B. Substitution of doctors by nurses in primary care. *Cochrane Database Syst Rev* 2005; (2): CD001271.

21. Banham L, Connelly J. Skill mix, doctors and nurses: substitution or diversification? *J Manag Med* 2002; **16**(4–5): 259–70.

22. Richardson G, Maynard A, Cullum N, Kindig D. Skill mix changes: substitution of service development? *Health Policy* 1998; **45**(2): 119–32.

23. Bunn F, Byrne G, Kendall S. telephone consultation and triage: effects on health care use and patient satisfaction *Cochrane Database Syst Rev* 2004; (4): CD004180.

24. Leese B, Allgar V, Heywood P, Walker R, Darr A, Din I, West RM. A new role for nurses as primary care cancer lead clinicians in Primary Care Trusts in England. *J Nurs Manage* 2006; **14**(6): 462–71.

25. Leese B. New opportunities for nurses and other healthcare professionals? A review of the potential impact of the new GMS contract on the primary care workforce. *J Health Organ Manage* 2006; **20**(6); 525–36.

26. Arie S. Can GPs compete with big business? *BMJ* 2006; 1172.

27. Holmes S, Gruffydd-Jones K, for the General Practice Airways group Education Sub-Committee. A proposal for the annual appraisal of, and developmental support for, General Practitioners with a specialist interest (GPwSIs) in respiratory medicine primary care. *Resp J* 2005; **14**(3): 161–5.

28. Moffat MA, Sheikh A, Price D, Peel A, Williams S, Cleland J, Pinnock M. Can a GP be a generalist and a specialist? Stakeholder views on a respiratory GP with a special interest service in the UK. *BMC Health Serv Res* 2006; **6**: 62.

29. Pinnock H, Netuveli G, Price D, Sheik A. General practitioners with a special interest in respiratory medicine: national survey of UK primary care organisations. *BMC Health Serv Res* 2005; **5**: 40.

30. Hay E, Campbell A, Linney S, Wise E, and on behalf of the Musculoskeletal GPwSI Working Group. Development of a competency framework for general practitioners with a special interest in musculoskeletal/rheumatology practice. *Rheumatology* 2007; **46**: 360–2.

31. Jones R, Rosen R, Tomlin Z, Cavanagh M-R, Oxley D. General practitioners with special interests: evolution and evaluation. *J Health Serv Res Policy* 2006; 11(2): 106–9.

32. Salusbury C, Noble A, Horrocks S, Crosby Z, Harrison V, Coast J. Evaluation of a general practitioners with special interest service for dermatology: randomised controlled trial. *BMJ* 2005; **331**: 1441–4.

33. Boggis A, Cornford C. General Practitioners with special interests: a qualitative study of the views of doctors, health managers and patients. *Health Policy* 2007; **80**: 172–8.

34. Bradley S, McKelvey DS. General practitioners with a special interest in public health; at last a way to deliver public health in primary care. *J Epidemiol Community Health* 2005; **59**(11): 920–3.

35. Coast J, Noble S, Noble A, Horrocks S, Asim O, Peters T, Salisbury C. Economic evaluation of a general practitioners with special interests led dermatology service in primary care. *BMJ* 2005; **331**: 1444–9.

36. Bodenheimer T, Wagner E, Grumbach K. Improving primary care for patients with chronic illness. *JAMA* 2002; **288**(14): 1775–9.

37. Department of Health. *Improving chronic disease management*. London: Department of Health, 2004.

38. Department of Health. *Supporting people with long term conditions: liberating the talents of nurses who care for people with long term conditions*. London: Department of Health, 2005.

39. Iliffe S, Gould MM, Wallace P. Assessment of older people in the community: lessons from Britain's '75 and over checks'. *Rev Clin Gerontol* 1999; **9**: 305–16.

40. Fletcher AE, Price GM, Ng ESW, Stirling SL, Breeze E, Bulpitt CJ, Nunes M, Jones DA, Latif A, Fasey NM, Vickers MR, Tulloch AJ. Population-based multidimensional assessment of older people in UK general practice: a cluster-randomised factorial trial. *Lancet* 2004; **364**: 1667–77.

41. Stuck AE, Beck JC, Egger M. Preventing disability in elderly people. *Lancet*; 2004; **364**: 1641–2.

42. Wagner E. Chronic disease management: what will it take to improve care for chronic illness? *Eff Clin Pract* 1998; **1**: 2–4.

43. Dixon J, Lewis R, Rosen R, Finalyson B, Gray D. *Managing chronic disease: What can we learn from the US experience?* London: Kings Fund Publications, 2004.

44. RCP, Royal College of General Practitioners and NHS Alliance. *Clinicians, services and commissioning in chronic disease management in the NHS; the need for co-ordinated management programmes.* London, 2004.

45. Drennan V, Goodman C. Primary Care Nurses and the use of case management for people with long-term conditions. *Br J Community Nurs* 2004; **9**(12): 22–6.

46. Wagner E, Davis C, Schaefer J, Von Korff M, Austin B. A survey of leading chronic disease management programs: are they consistent with the literature? *J Nurs Care Qual* 2002; **16**(2): 67–80.

47. Drennan V, Iliffe S, Hanworth D, See Tai S, Lenihan P, Deave T. A picture of health. *Health Serv J* 2003; **113**(5852): 22–4.

48. De Lepeleire J, Heyrman J. Is everyone with a chronic disease also chronically ill? *Arch Public Health* 2003; **61**: 161–76.

49. Roland M, Dusheiko M, Gravelle H, Parker S. Follow up of people aged 65 and over with a history of emergency admissions: analysis of routine admission data. *BMJ* 2005; **330**(7486): 289–92.

50. Cullum N, Spilsbury K, Richardson G. Nurse led care. *BMJ* 2005; **330**(7493): 682–3.

51. Boadenheimer T, Macgregor K, Stodart N. Nurses as leaders in chronic care. *BMJ* 2005; **330**: 612–13.

52. Royal College of Nursing and Royal College of General Practice. Report of the Joint Working Party on the primary health care team. London: RGCP, 1961.

53. Department of Health and Social Security. The Primary Health Care Team Report of the Joint Working Group of the Standing Medical Advisory Committee and the Standing Nursing and Midwifery Committee (Chairman W. Harding). London: DHSS, 1981.

54. Abel R. Staff implications of schemes of attachment of Local Health Authority staff (HV and Home Nursing) to General Practitioners. Study No.1 1969 DHSS Social Science Research Unit. London: HMSO.

55. Department of Health and Social Security. *Neighbourhood nursing—a focus for care.* London: HMSO, 1986.

56. Marsh G, Kaim Caudle P. *Teamwork in general practice.* London: Croom-Helm, 1976.

57. Gregson B, *et al. Interprofessional collaboration in primary health care organisations.* Occasional Paper 52. London: Royal College of General Practitioners, 1991.

58. Audit Commission. *Homeward bound.* London: Audit Commission, 1992.

59. Koperski M *et al.* Nurse practitioners in general practice an inevitable progression? *Br J Gen Pract* 1997; 696–7.

60. Editorial. The latest official statistics. *Employing Nurses* 1996; September: 10–11.

61. Green S. A pivot for the practice. *Nurs Times* 1993; **89**: 46 42–4.

62. Knott M. Integrated nursing teams: developments in general practice. *Community Pract* 1999; **72**(2): 23–4.

63. The NHS and Community Care Act 1990. London: HMSO, 1990.

64. Department of Health NHS Modern and Dependable (Cm. 3852). London: The Stationery Office, 1998.

65. Pearson P, Jones K. Primary care—opportunities and threats. *BMJ* 1997; **314**(7083): 817–20.

66. Firth-Cozens J. Celebrating teamwork. *Qual Health Care* 1998; 7 (Suppl.) S3–7.

67. Royal Pharmaceutical Society of Great Britain, BMA. *Teamworking in primary health care: realising shared aims in patient care.* London: Royal Pharmaceutical Society of Great Britain, the British Medical Association, 2000.

68. Royal College of General Practitioners. *The nature of general medical practice.* Report from General Practice, No. 27. London: Royal College of General Practitioners, 1996.

69. Poulton B, West M. The determinant of effectiveness in multi-disciplinary teamwork in primary health care. *Journal of Interprofessional Care*, 1999; **13**(1): 7–18.

70. Gregson *et al.* 1991 op cit.

71. Kharicha K, Iliffe S, Levin E, Davey B, Fleming C. Tearing down the Berlin Wall: social workers' perspectives on joint working with general practice. *Fam Pract* 2005; **22**: 399–405.

72. Huntingdon J. *Social work and general medical practice.* London: George Allen and Unwin, 1981.

73. Ovretveit J. Essentials of multidisciplinary organisation. Uxbridge: Brunel University, 1988.

74. See, for example, Gregson *et al.* 1991 *Op cit.*

75. Pritchard P. In *Inter-professional issues in community and primary health care.* Owens P, *et al.* (eds). London: Macmillan Press, 1995.

76. Pearson-P, Jones-K. Primary care—opportunities and threats. *BMJ* 1997; **314**(7083): 817–20.

77. Kharicha K, Levin E, Iliffe S, Davey B. Tearing down the Berlin Wall: social work, general practice and evidence based policy in the collaborative care of older people. *Health Soc Care Community* 2004; **12**(2): 134–41.

78. Firth-Cozens J 1998 *op cit.*

79. Sennett R. *The corrosion of character*. London: Norton, 1998, p. 110.

80. United States Department of Labor. *What work requires of schools: a SCANS report for America 2000*. Washington DC: United States Department of Labor, 1991.

81. Graham L. *On the line at Subaru-Isuzu*. Ithica, NY: Cornell University Press, 1995, p. 108.

82. Kunda G. *Engineering culture: control and commitment in a high-tech corporation*. Philadelphia, PA: Temple University Press, 1992, p. 156.

83. Sennett R. *The corrosion of character*. London: Norton, 1998, p. 112.

84. Roberts VZ. The self-assigned impossible task. In *The unconscious at work: individual and organisational stress in the human services*. Obholzer A, Roberts VZ (eds). London: Routledge, 1994, pp. 112–15.

85. Miller C, Freeman M, Ross N. *Interprofessional practice in health and social care: challenging the shared learining agenda*. London: Arnold, 2001.

86. Centre for the Advancement of Interprofessional Education Interprofessional education: a definition. *CAIPE Bull* 1997; **13**: 19.

87. Lavin M, Ruebling I. Interdisciplinary health professional education: a historical review. *Adv Health Sci Educ* 2001; **6**: 25–47.

88. Hackman J. *Groups that work (and those that don't)*. California: Jossey-Bass, 1990.

89. West M. *Effective teamworking*. London: Sage, 1994.

90. West M, Poulton B. Primary care teams: in a league of their own. In *Promoting teamwork in primary care*. Pearson P, Spencer J (eds). London: Arnold, 1997.

91. Sheard A, Kakabadse A. A process perspective on leadership and team development. *J Manage Dev* 2004; **23**: 7–106.

92. Toner J, Miller P, Gurland J. Conceptual, theoretical and practical approaches to the development of interdisciplinary teams: a transactional model. *Educ Gerontol* 1994; **20**: 53–69.

93. Payne M. *Teamwork in multiprofessional care*. Basingstoke: Palgrave, 2000.

94. Ovretveit J. How to describe interprofessional working. In *Interprofessional working for health and social care*. Oevreitveit J, Mathias P, Thompson T (eds). Basingstoke: MacMillan Press, 1997.

95. Southon G, Braithwaite J. *The end of professionalism*. In *Changing practice in health and social care*. Davies C, Finlay L, Bullman A (eds). London: Sage, 2000.

96. Engel C. A functional anatomy of teamwork. In *Going interprofessional: working together for health and welfare*. Leatherard A (ed.). London: Routledge, 1994.

97. Sennett R. *The corrosion of character*. London: Norton, 1998, p. 114.

98. Rorty R. *Contingency, irony and solidarity*. Cambridge: Cambridge University Press, 1989, pp. 73–91.

99. Sennett R. *The corrosion of character*. London: Norton, 1998, p. 117.

100. Coser L. *The functions of social conflict*. New York: Free Press, 1976.

101. Gutman A, Thompson D. *Democracy and disagreement*. Cambridge, MA: Harvard University Press, 1996.

102. Heath I, Sweeney K. Medical generalists: connecting the map and the territory. *BMJ* 2005: **331**: 1462–4.

103. Tudor Hart J. *A new kind of doctor*. London: Merlin 1988.

104. Giddens A. *Modernity, self identity: self and society in the late modern age*. Cambridge: Polity Press, 2002, p. 31.

105. Godsen T, Forland F, Kristiansen I, *et al*. Capitation, salary, fee-for-service and mixed systems of payment: effects on the behaviour of primary care physicians. *Cochrane Database Systematic Rev* 2000; **3**: CD002215.

106. Sorensen R, Grytten J. Service production and contract choice in primary physician services. *Health Policy* 2003; **66**: 73–93.

107. Gosden T, Sibbald B, Williams J, Petchey R, Leese B. Paying doctors by salary: a controlled study of general practitioner behaviour in England. *Health Policy* 2003; **64**(3): 415–23.

108. Gosden T, Foreland F, Kristiansen I, Sutton M, Leese B, Giuffrida A, Sergison M, Pedersen L. Impact of payment method on behaviour of primary care physicians: a systematic review. *J Health Serv Res Policy* 2001.

109. Giuffrida A, Gosden T, Forland F, Kristiansen I, Sergison M, Leese B, Pedersen L, Sutton M. Target payments in primary care: effects on professional practice and health care outcomes. *Cochrane Database Syst Rev* 2000; (3): CD000531.

110. Sorensen R, Grytten J. Contract design for primary care physicians: physical location and practice behaviour in small communities. *Health Care Manage Sci* 2000; **3**(2): 151–7.

Chapter 4

Mass production

State-driven clinical priorities are risking
general practice's disciplinary identity. By
allowing ourselves to be coerced into persuading
patients to follow particular treatments in
return for financial gain, we risk further losing
our professional identity and reputation. More
importantly, the very presence of the (quality
outcomes) framework is deeply corrosive to the
ethical practice of medicine.
Dee Mangin & Les Toop BJGP (June 2007)[1]

Assembling the optimal range of disciplines within primary care is
one task, and ensuring a standard level of quality services is another.
It is not enough to know that a range of different skills is being
applied to meet the range of needs in a local population; the local
health service management also needs to know that the quality of
care is both good and uniform across the locality, and that mechanisms for continuously monitoring of that quality are both in place
and in routine use. In the name of equity the National Health Service's
(NHS) leadership needs to assure its Ministers that the same standard
of care is available in every area, regardless of the peculiarities of the
area. A citizen should get the same effective treatment in general practice for otitis media, chronic obstructive pulmonary disease, chest
pain, depression, shingles, or any other common problem or condition that could be managed within the community in Bradford as
they would receive in Bridlington, even if the service is delivered in a
different language in each place.

This political objective is a just one, and one that motivates many in
medicine, but it is also one that requires a degree of uniformity in

clinical work that challenges the individual, highly tailored approach that some say is a defining feature of general practice. It shifts the focus from the individuality of the patient, and the complex ways in which personality, experience, and resilience interact to produce an illness, to the similarities of disease in different people and the common effect it has on a diverse range of characters. The doctor or nurse then spends less time understanding or experiencing the perspective of the patient and more time in trying to change it where it diverges from the medical model, and reinforce it where it converges.

From craft work to mass production

The practical problems for those reshaping general practice and engineering forward integration are fourfold. First, diagnoses need to be made according to accepted protocols or using standardized classification systems. Heart failure then becomes a diagnosis that is reached only by interpretation of symptoms in the light of the results of an echocardiogram, while depression requires the use of a standardized instrument, validated for use in community settings, which distinguishes 'true' depression from unhappiness, and then categorizes it by severity.

Second, treatments initiated in response to the diagnosis should be drawn from an approved formulary of drugs or battery of non-drug treatments, all of which have been shown to have demonstrable, unarguable positive effects at a price that is acceptable to the architects of an integrated health service. Treatments can be allocated to different categories of effectiveness, using the methods of evidence-based medicine that we will come to in Chapter 5, by experts in their use, who can weight the clinical value and the costs of one treatment against another.

Third, referral from general practice to specialist services should occur for the same kinds of problems in different places, although availability of resources may erode equitable provision. There must be, then, criteria that should be met before referral occurs, and individual patients must be eligible for specialist services. Some mechanism for reviewing the appropriateness of referrals, and their concordance with referral criteria, is therefore needed.

Four, knowing that the quality of the continuing medical management of long-term conditions in general practice is sustained at a high level requires monitoring of processes. This monitoring should accommodate overlapping conditions or co-morbidities, so that (for example) the presence and impact of depression is assessed in any patient with a long-term medical condition or disability, and acted upon.

If these problems can be overcome, high-quality and standardized care in general practice could be achieved through the micro-management of consultations. If the thinking and actions of doctors can be prescribed by the NHS across a range of clinical problems, their diagnostic and treatment decisions, referral patterns and management systems could be shaped into a coherent and consistent process. The micro-management of the consultation, if achievable, could bring general practitioners (GPs) under the same sort of control as a salaried employee without actually making them salaried. This ambition corresponds to Richard Sennett's *Disc World* method of management at a distance, and echoes Foucault's ideas about exerting power and imposing discipline through surveillance. Sennett argues that modern organizations are structured like CD players, with a central processing unit that scans information on the disc.[2] No intervening layers of management can modify or re-organize the data—there is no 'interpretive modulation'—and the central processing unit can see clearly and exactly what is happening by what the data shows. In the days of the primary care group GPs and other primary care professionals could influence the debates within the administrative structures of the health service, the thinking that guided them and the decisions that they took and implemented. The Primary Care Groups were 'interpretive modulators' between the professionals and the Department of Health. Their replacement by larger Primary Care Trusts (PCTs) that were less open to professional influence reduced that interpretive modulation, taking the organization of general practice a step nearer to Sennett's Disc management model. Now a 'central processing' unit can read the data collected on practice systems directly, observing the practices achieve the targets of the Quality Outcomes Framework (QOF).

Objections to mass production

We could resist the efforts to insinuate a new industrial discipline into general practice on a number of grounds. Constructing medicine in terms of diagnoses, treatments, referral, and long-term management is not congruent with much of what we do in general practice, our work being less linear and algorithmic and more messy and uncertain, with containment of anxiety a major (but hard to measure) component. It could be, in effect, the colonization of generalism's wide perspectives by the narrow logic of specialist practice. We try to change the explanatory models of health and illness in our patients, so that they do not think that subjective wellness means immunity from illness, that unprotected sex is risk-free or that hazardous behaviour carries no penalties, but we try to tailor it to their individual perceptions and understanding. Mass production in general practice using a specialist framework of thinking can be seen as a similar process, with our explanatory models being replaced by others created in the very different environment of the hospital. Faced with a depressed patient, we are encouraged (by financial inducements) to measure the breadth and depth of their depression using standard instruments, the PHQ9 or the Hospital Anxiety & Depression (HAD) scale. Even if they are not obviously depressed, but have diabetes or heart disease, we are encouraged to ask screening questions to unmask depressive symptoms that can then be assessed using the fuller instruments. These are potentially useful steps, but taking them leads us into difficult areas, because the linear logic of the diagnostic process excludes the person's context and biography, and side-steps all controversy about what 'depression' really is. Dougal Jeffries captured the incongruence between the diagnostic logic of the specialist who has been condensed into a rating scale and the usual GP bespoke approach of 'attentive listening, some problem-solving suggestions, referral for counselling or psychotherapy and the use of medication.'[3] Having abandoned the use of HAD because it distracted him from these actions while not altering his clinical management, he was appalled by the financial inducement to use it (or a specified equivalent) in the QOF, noted the weakness of the evidence that use of the scales alters outcomes for patients (other than surrogate ones of being categorized), and chastized the 'Department of Health, the pharmaceutical industry, and their academic comrades-in-arms' for subverting general practice. This is a substantive issue, with the issues of recognizing depression being explored by Chris Dowrick in his book

Beyond depression,[4] while Charles Medawar has called the somewhat collusive construction of depression as a diagnostic category by psychiatrists and the pharmaceutical industry a 'conspiracy of goodwill'.[5]

These arguments add up to a plausible objection to the processes of mass production, in my view, but not entirely convincing one. The micro-management of the consultation can only occur when there are easily measured activities and aspects of practice that are easy to quantify. These activities—giving smoking cessation advice, reducing blood pressure, monitoring renal function and reacting to renal failure—are ones where a structured approach is helpful to the practitioner as well as to the patient. The QOF may well be rewarding efforts at improving surrogate outcomes such as blood pressure control, cholesterol levels, and HbA1c measures, but we have good enough grounds for thinking these are worthwhile objectives. This may even be true of depression, which as a clinical condition is at the outer limits of the medical model. We should note the evidence that screening for depression may not be beneficial to our patients,[6] and we should be sceptical about the academic industry that forever seeks the elusive brief diagnostic instrument that will transform general practice, the perfect spanner that will unlock and simplify complexities. There is much reductionist thinking in specialist medicine, and academia is sometimes divorced from practice and often self-absorbed, but we should not underestimate the limitations of generalism. The transition from novice GP to expert occurs over a long period of time in which skills are accumulated. I suspect Dougal Jeffries abandoned HAD because it was not complex enough for him, but in using it he may well have incorporated some of its logic and structure into his own, more complex, way of thinking about depression. The new GP joining their practice, on the other hand, may have a less complex model of depression, and would benefit professionally from using HAD. The deployment of diagnostic tools such as HAD with the QOF tells us that some powerful body sees general practice as underskilled, a view that we would need to challenge with hard evidence if we wanted to delete the use of depression scales from the package of targets. We might be better off if we accept that the organization of clinical work using information technologies to regulate processes of investigation, treatment and assessment frees time and effort for the complex, messy, and fuzzy parts of clinical activity, which will continue to demand our attention. Generalism could be strengthened rather than weakened by the incorporation of linear, algorithmic thinking, which cannot be claimed by specialists as their kind of knowledge, but rather is a common substrate for all clinical practice. The task for general practice is to avoid being overwhelmed by reductionist thinking, but still to use its products. Postgraduate training in general practice is highly developed, and reflects the complexity and richness of generalist practice and thinking. We can be reasonably confident that, over time, this system of professional development will continue to undo some of the intellectual distortion induced by experience of hospital medicine. In other words, we do have a mechanism, however flawed, that could help replicate Dougal Jeffries' expertise while also fostering his style of critical thinking.

We could object to the loss of autonomy that micro-management of the consultation requires, but it may be worth experiencing. Codified good practice is still good practice, as long as there is a consensus about its provenance, and constitutes the rule system needed if we want to apply an evolving medical science to individuals and populations. As Martin Roland points out, the QOF depends in large part on professional judgements about the importance of different aspects of clinical care, and this is no bad thing.[7] Autonomy in this situation should be the kind of clinical freedom that is the recognition of necessity. When autonomy is defined operationally as the right of individual practitioners to prioritize which aspects of medicine they wish to apply in their practice, the results are unacceptable variations in provision that voluntary collaborations, appeals to professional ethics and even the provision of extra resources cannot entirely abolish.

I think that most of us are likely to be comfortable with this incorporation of structured care as long as it manageable within restraints of routine consultations, or delegatable to other staff. Mass production styles of working are nothing new in general practice, which has a high turnover form of consultation into which ever more activity is being introduced. We may not have to work at the pace of the early days of NHS general practice, with 40 patients in morning and evening surgeries and a dozen house calls in between, and we are no longer reduced to the kind of advice a veteran GP in my area once gave about patient management to an incoming doctor—'don't let them sit down'—but the consultations are now so full with differing agendas that notices urging patients not to bring lists seem commonplace in waiting rooms. As we have seen, GPs work more readily with clearly defined conditions such as heart disease than with more diffuse problems like mental illness. Despite the sustained efforts of the Royal College of General Practitioners over decades, we are still better equipped to work in the 'bio' component of the biopsychosocial model of generalism than we are in the psychological or social domains. Finally, as we have also already seen, general practice remains a subaltern discipline in the power hierarchy of medicine, and is therefore likely to adopt the thinking and ways of working of the dominant model. Measuring thyroid function makes sense to us in a way that taking a detailed occupational history, assessing the level of carer strain or mapping explanatory models do not.

Knaves or knights?

Another objection to the micro-management of the consultation is that the linkage of concordance with guidelines with payment may give the pursuit of quality something of a 'bonus' status, not a professionally endorsed moral good. This may be true as long as the incentives to provide quality care—as defined by concordance with guidelines—are a small component of the practice economy. The moment the balance between quality payments and payments for dealing with complex and messy demands shift to give a decisive economic weight to quality, the risks of underperformance matter. Whatever we might like to think about the professionalism of our discipline, the behaviour of GPs as a whole corresponds more to that of knaves than of knights, in the sense that we are driven by the local economy of the practice (and the surrounding NHS) as much as if not more than by a sense of professionalism. The evidence for this is disparate but in my view convincing enough to explain the approach taken by the Department of Health towards refining the GP contract since 1997. For example, early analysis of the factors promoting development in general practice by Bosanquet and Leese[8] suggested that it depended on rising list sizes, brown-field sites for new buildings and the ready availability of low-cost ancillary staff, with professional leadership playing a dominant role mainly in inner-city areas where these economic conditions did not necessarily apply.

If economic factors outweigh professional imperatives in shaping our behaviour, there are risks to the health service and to the public from GPs 'gaming' the system of financial rewards to maximize practice income. Bevan and Hood describe how gaming has occurred in hospitals,[9] but the same processes are likely to apply in general practice. There are three main risks:

1. **Poor performance in domains where performance is not measured**. For example, the effort put into influenza immunization may detract attention from the case management of older patients with multiple comorbidities, making it necessary to employ 'community matrons' to pick up this task.

2. **Hitting the target but missing the point**. For example, pressure to reduce referrals means that appropriate referrals are delayed or not made at all, particularly if patient ambivalence is powerful, as is sometimes the case with investigation and treatment of remediable eye diseases, joint replacement, or treatment of urinary incontinence.

3. **Discrepancies in data recording**. For example, blood pressure measurements that do not fit below the target thresholds may not be documented, or put in free text, or even altered to conform and achieve the target level.

The same problems can arise in general practice, with practitioners being accused of manipulating prevalence data to boost pay and reporting patients as exceptions inappropriately.[10] While Bevan and Hood argue that 'systems need to be put in place to minimise gaming to meet targets and to ensure targets are not causing unwanted effects elsewhere', it is difficult to see what such 'systems' might be and reasonable to wonder whether it might be better not to have reimbursable targets at all, or at least not to make them so central to the practice economy.

Social consequences

A final objection to the industrialization of practice and the intrusion of mass production techniques into at least some parts of the consultation is that the new focus on achievable processes and out-comes will crowd out the more humanistic elements of clinical work, to do with the containment of psychopathology or the amelioration of misery. We will be too busy attending to the pop-ups in the corner of the screen to pay attention to the stories that are being told to us, and to unravelling their meaning. GPs could become preoccupied with the anatomical dissection of clinical process, limiting their abil-ity to respond to wider issues. Getting the number of medication reviews right might well have some beneficial if mostly modest long-term effects on patient health, but the downsizing of the local physio-therapy or district nursing team by a cash-strapped PCT is likely to have more immediate and potentially more costly consequences to patients, their families, and the health service. Similarly, skills acquired in managing surrogate outcomes may absorb the time and effort needed to develop attentive listening, apply cognitive-behavioural therapy-based containment techniques with patients with recurring problems of adaptation to the demands of work and relationships, or respond to consumerist challenges.

The consequences could be significant, because containment of psychopathology is essential for social cohesion and the legitimiza-tion of the existing order as the best of all possible worlds, or perhaps as the least worst. If it is crowded out by preoccupations with the technically measurable those feeling ignored or unsupported may reduce their support for the current pattern of social relationships. The quality of public services, of which health services are a major subsystem, offers the basis for trust in the state, without which gov-ernments lack the political legitimacy to govern.[11] The risk is not that a disgruntled patient population would rise up and overthrow the government but rather that it might invest its interest and money in commercialized medicine in all its forms, from traditional private practice to High Street homeopaths and acupuncturists. At the level of the individual this does not much matter, and we may think it entirely appropriate (or perhaps even experience relief) if some peo-ple transferred their allegiance to colonic irrigators and reflexologists. At a societal level it may matter more, if the transfer of allegiance leads to an emotional and political disinvestment from allopathy as a whole, from the NHS as an institution and from general practice as the embodiment of family medicine. We will return to this issue in Chapter 7.

Incentives to improve quality

There is no one mechanism for overcoming barriers to change in healthcare and for re-configuring services, everything being contingent on history and setting.[12] Conscious attempts to produce changes in professional behaviour, therefore, tend to be experimental and incremental, without a master plan to which all parties must adhere. Methods for altering clinical practice are tried out, discarded if ineffective, relegated to minor roles if weakly effective, or subsumed within more complex policies if they show signs of success. One consequence of this trial and error approach to policy implementation is the appearance and disappearance of different 'brands' of thinking, with health improvement programmes and total quality management coming and going while National Service Frameworks arrive and stay (for the moment). Another is that requirements that GPs must meet can change almost as fast as we learn how to do them, and probably at an even faster pace than evolving treatment regimens. For example, the unilateral imposition of a new contract for general practice that began the industrialization process in 1990 sought to incentivize health promotion by focusing on identifying patients with risks, rather than documenting interventions or recording outcomes. There was then some evidence of perverse incentives operating, with less activity occurring in areas of greatest need,[13] and as the QOF measures similar surrogate outcomes we should expect the same pattern—the best organized practices, which are disproportionately represented in the areas of lower need, will do best.

Whatever the inequities in the impact of these incentives to change practice, there are some grounds for thinking that they will work. Even before the incentives built into the 2004 contract could make a difference on clinical practice there were measurable reductions in the number of hospital admissions for acute and chronic conditions manageable in primary care, over the period between 1998 and 2003.[14] The changing pattern of outcomes from stroke is illuminating because stroke's major risk factor—hypertension—is the focus of so much attention in general practice. Although the prevalence of hypertension had not changed over this time period, the proportions of those with treated and controlled hypertension had risen. There was a significant fall in the population levels of hospital admission for stroke, despite the expectation that newly developed stroke units would increase admission rates. Case fatality and population mortality for stroke both fell, and timely discharge to usual place of residence after stroke increased significantly. The quality of primary care, particularly around hypertension management, is likely to be one of the factors shaping these trends, alongside local population characteristics and the way outpatient and inpatient services operate. Forward integration of primary and secondary care does appear to have had an impact on disease management, with effects accumulating over a relatively short time period. GPs see the rationale behind the incentives package and do not identify the quality and outcomes framework as a major assault on their autonomy, at least in an early and admittedly small study.[15]

There are negative experiences too. The UK was the first country to introduce a nationwide screening programme for older citizens without plausible evidence of health gain, and has been followed by others in Europe mesmerized by perceptions of the rising demographic tide.[16] The '75 and over checks' were introduced in 1990, despite the objections of family doctors, and in practice were widely ignored. Undoubtedly the lack of a credible evidence base, and the lack of guidance on how to carry out the 75 and over assessments added to their unpopularity with GPs, and led to piecemeal and often unenthusiastic implementation of the programme.[17] Where assessment tasks were undertaken at all they were delegated to practice nurses and were given low priority by the local health service administration[18] that (with a few exceptions) provided neither leadership nor training for the programme, nor policed its implementation.

Testing incentive packages

The lessons that seemed to have been learned by the Department of Health from early efforts to standardize clinical practice were that incentives had to focus on process measures (performance indicators), that micro-management of clinical work could reach into the consultation (specifying some of its content), that protocols, guidelines, and pathways should be available for as many domains of clinical care as possible, and that clinical activity should be audited regularly. These lessons were put into operation in 2004, in the QOF. QOF translates nationally determined clinical priorities into tasks to be carried out in encounters with patients, and relies upon automated auditing of performance not only to measure the quality of care, but also to reward it. However, before performance indicators were implemented through a contract they were tested in practice, a departure from the earlier, much cruder approaches to industrialization in 1990.

Although the use of performance indicators in the public sector was a feature of the New Public Management of the 1980s, and therefore preceded the overt industrialization of the general practice, most of the learning about the impact of performance indicators in clinical settings followed the first attempts to standardize practice, in the 1990 contract. Performance indicators challenge a usually well-guarded aspect of professional autonomy, the assessment of work performance. Studies of GPs' responses to the introduction of performance indicators revealed how practitioners' thinking about their work was changing. Five themes seemed to sum up GPs' responses: (1) the credibility of the performance indicators; (2) the acceptance that competence needed to be demonstrated; (3) ambivalence about autonomy; (4) the ulterior purpose of performance indicators; and (5) the identity of the assessor of performance.[19]

Performance indicators need to be sensible and important to clinical practice, if they are to be accepted. GPs discussing them in the study by Exworthy and colleagues[19] were concerned that performance indicators could not capture the reality of generalism, in particular consultation skills, continuity of care, and the 'pastoral' work of ongoing support that enhanced the quality of life of some patients. There was a sense that general practice as a discipline defied analysis, and even that it was inherently unscientific, making performance indicators into inadequate or false measures of performance and competence, especially when there were shifting thresholds for interventions (as, for example, in hyperlipidaemia) or swings in therapeutic fashion, as around cut-off values for hypertension treatment.

What was very striking was the acceptance by GPs that competence needed to be demonstrated. This fits with the historic redefinition of professionalism described by Marquand (see Chapter 1) as being less to do with acting in the public good and more to do with having special knowledge and expertise. Acts in the public good are by definition public, whereas special knowledge and skills have to be exposed, even excavated, to reveal the actual as opposed to proclaimed competence of the practitioner. This shift in thinking about external assessment may be one reason why resistance to the 2004 new General Medical Services contract was more muted than to the 1990 contract. Equally striking was the ambivalence felt about autonomy, which was seen as under threat in a general sense while also not specifically threatened by sensible clinical indicators that autonomous professionals should be using already. It was the ulterior purpose of performance indicators that undermined any sense of security, as they were seen as sticks to accompany the carrots of contract change, and precursors to more stringent government interference in clinical practice.

Finally, in the Exworthy study the identity of the assessor determined the response that GPs made to the assessment of their work. Physically distant assessors were acceptable as long as they shared expertise, collegiality, and identity with general practice. Ceding control of assessment to superordinate GPs (in management roles in PCTs), academic GPs or public health doctors was an acceptable compromise that preserved some level of autonomy by placing a general practice friendly mediator (Sennett's 'interpretive modulators') between data captured from the desktop PC and the general managers of the NHS.

Performance indicators

In these early studies the most common response to the introduction of performance indicators in general practice was to improve data quality through increased or improved accuracy of recording. There was, however, a lack of co-ordinated team approach to decision-making about meeting performance indicators, and little interest in their use as a tool to address inequalities between practices.[20] The potential of performance indicators as measures of quality of care needed further research, according to the academics,[21] but the government had the intelligence it needed and did not wait, opting instead to implement QOF. The negotiations between the State and the discipline's leaders were not acrimonious, as in 1990, and when the 2004 contract rewarded practices financially there was no dousing of militancy by prosperity, because there was little or no militancy to douse.

The critics of mass production methods in medicine, and of their importation into general practice, may be right about the scale of their impact on the discipline, in the sense that organizationally based performance indicators may end the detachment of general practice from the main body of the NHS. They could draw us so deeply into the public domain that we come very close to entering the public sector. Sennett's Disc World may well be coming into being, with the 'central processing unit' scanning the data on the hard drive of every practice's server. Our information technology—with the electronic patient record at its centre—is crucial in revealing how GPs perform, and the computer on the desk becomes a window on to clinical practice, but one which can transmit, conceal, or distort different aspects of clinical work. It all depends on who looks through it and for what purpose.[19] One type of conflict that seems likely to develop within primary care will be around who audits whom.

Audit

As David Marquand points out, one of the problems with audit is that it is an iron cage. At the same time audits produce assurance or increased confidence in the subject matter of audit[22]—in this case the quality of GP care. Professional activities are necessarily opaque and mysterious to outsiders, making it difficult for outsiders to measure quality, in the sense of the qualities of the good doctor. External audit then requires proxy measures of quality, in quantitative form, but it has proved easy to pick unhelpful audit criteria and so measure the wrong things.[23] This problem has exercised the collective mind of the National Institute for Health & Clinical Excellence, which now attempts to select audit criteria as rigorously as it sieves evidence for guidelines, and it will continue to exercise the minds of practitioners, at practice and PCT levels.

Once professionals are subject to external audit of quantitative proxy measures, their practices get altered to fit the audit requirements and their room for interpretation—their autonomy—declines, while local structures of trust between auditors (in PCTs) and the audited in practices may be displaced and potentially distorted.[24] The avoidance of this risk has been one of the concerns that appears to have influenced the formulation and implementation of the new 2004 General Medical Services contract, and the Department of Health has relied upon the entry of GPs into management as a way of fitting proxy measures as closely as possible with clinical realities.

If who audits whom is the issue for general practice, we might decide to develop audit skills and become the auditors, both of ourselves and of those who manage local health services. Given that command philosophies of regulation are giving way to forms of control that utilize the resources of the regulatee,[25] this will in principle fit neatly into the industrialization of general practice. In practice it may be very different, as a significant proportion of GPs may be unable to adequately apply audit methods, raising serious questions about the effectiveness of clinical audit as a healthcare improvement policy for general practice.[26]

Micro-managing the consultation

How far can and should the micro-management of the consultation go? There are risks in making GPs into demotivated data collectors. Professor Chris Ham emphasizes the importance of professional commitment:

> Fixing the problems of the NHS requires shifting from a culture of compliance with externally imposed targets to a culture of commitment in which the principled motivation of staff is leveraged to deliver improvements for patients ... This requires every NHS organization to give priority to engaging doctors and other clinicians in the next stage of the journey of reform.[27]

Jennifer Dixon, Director of Policy at the King's Fund, is clear about what needs to be done with general practice.[28] First, the 'principle of introducing new incentives to try and improve performance is the right one'. Second, the lack of 'contractual obligations for GPs to manage the resources they are spending and influencing on behalf of their patients' is a problem that needs to be remedied by sanctioning GPs for not commissioning services, or for doing so badly.

By contrast, Northumberland GP Steven Ford proposes that 'Simplicity, delegation and non-interference will yield the prize' and that a 'coherent, locally responsive service, answerable to users directly is preferable to a national business failure with a demoralised workforce. Let diversity flourish and to hell with the market.'[29]

Notions of professionalism, accountability and autonomy continue to compete for our attention, seemingly in contradiction to one another. The resolution of these contradictions is the next task for the management of the NHS, in debate with the profession, as it searches for a powerful intellectual glue that will hold an industrializing discipline together. In Chapters 5 and 6 we will examine the glues on offer, evidence-based medicine and clinical governance.

References

1. Mangin D, Toop L. The Quality and Outcomes Framework: what have you done to yourselves? *Br J Gen Pract* 2007: **57**: 435–7.
2. Sennett R. *Respect: the formation of character in an age of inequality*. London: Penguin Books, 2004.
3. Jeffries D. Ever been HAD? *Br J Gen Pract* 2006; **56**: 392.
4. Dowrick C. *Beyond depression*. Oxford: Oxford University Press, 2004.
5. Medawar C. *Medicines out of control: antidepressants and the conspiracy of goodwill*. Amsterdam: Aksant Academic Publishers 2004.
6. Gilbody S, Sheldon T, Wessley S. Should we screen for depression? *BMJ* 2006; **332**: 1027–30.
7. Roland M. The Quality and Outcomes Framework: too early for a final verdict. *Br J Gen Pract* 2007; **57**: 525–7.
8. Bosanquet N, Leese B. Family doctors and innovation in general practice. *BMJ* 1988; **296**: 1576–80.
9. Bevan G, Hood C. Have targets improved performance in the English NHS? *BMJ* 2006; **332**: 419–22.
10. Rigby J. Practices hit by QOF gaming accusations. *Pulse*, 2007; **7 June**.
11. Thompson A. New millennium, new values: citizen participation as the democratic ideal in health care. *Int J Qual Health Care* 1999; **11**(6): 461–4.
12. Shaw B, Cheater F, Baker R, Gillies C, Hearnshaw H, Flottorp S, Robertson N. Tailored interventions to overcome identified barriers to change: effects on professional practice and health care outcomes. *Cochrane Database Syst Rev* 2005; (3): CD005470.
13. Langham S, Gillam S, Thorogood M. The carrot, the stick and the general practitioner: how have changes in financial incentives affected health promotion in general practice? *Br J Gen Pract* 1995; **45**: 665–8.

14. Lakhani A, Coles J, Eayres D, Spence C, Rachet B. Creative use of existing clinical and health outcomes data to assess NHS performance in England: Part 1—performance indicators closely linked to clinical care. *BMJ* 2005: **330**: 1426–31.

15. McDonald R, Harrison S, Checkland K, Campbell S, Roland M. Impact of financial incentives on clinical autonomy and internal motivation in primary care: ethnographic study. *BMJ* 2007; **334**: 1357–9.

16. Bernabei R, Landi F, Gambassi G, *et al.* Randomised trial of impact of model of integrated care and case management for older people living in community. *BMJ* 1998; **316**: 1348–51.

17. Brown, K, Williams E, Groom L. Health checks on patients 75 years and over in Nottinghamshire after the new GP contract *BMJ* 1992; **305**: 619–21.

18. Chew CA, Wilkin D, Glendinning C. Annual assessments of patients aged 75 years and over: general practitioners' and nurses' views and experience. *Br J Gen Pract* 1994; **44**: 263–7.

19. Exworthy M, Wlkinson E, McColl A, Moore M, Roderick P, Smith H, Gabbay J. The role of performance indicators in changing the autonomy of the general practice profession in the UK. *Soc Sci Med* 2003; **56**: 1493–504.

20. Wilkinson E, McColl A, Exworthy M, Roderick P, Smith H, Moore M, Gabbay J. Reactions to the use of evidence-based performance indicators in primary care: a qualitative study. *Qual Health Care* 2000; **9**: 166–74.

21. McColl A, Roderick P, Wilkinson E, Gabbay J, Smith H, Moore M, Exworthy M. Clinical governance in primary care groups: the feasibility of deriving evidence-based performance indicators. *Qual Health Care* 2000; **9**: 90–7.

22. Power M. Auditing and the production of legitimacy. *Accounting Organ Soc* 2003; **28**: 379–94.

23. Hearnshaw H, Harker R, Cheater F, Baker R, Grimshaw G. Are audits wasting resources by measuring the wrong things? A survey of methods used to select audit review criteria. *Qual Saf Health Care* 2003; **12**: 24–8.

24. Marquand D. *Decline of the public*. Cambridge: Polity Press, 2004, p. 111.

25. Power M. Expertise and the construction of relevance: accountants and environmental audit. *Accounting Organ Soc* 1997; **22**(2): 123–46.

26. McKay J, Bowie P, Lough M. Variations in the ability of general medical practitioners to apply two methods of clinical audit: a five year study of assessment by peer review. *J Eval Clin Pract* 2006; **12**(6): 622–9.

27. Quoted in: Kmietowicz Z. One year to save the NHS: what would you do? *BMJ* 2007; **334**: 181.

28. Quoted in: Kmietowicz Z. One year to save the NHS: what would you do? *BMJ* 2007; **334**: 180–181.

29. Quoted in: Kmietowicz Z. One year to save the NHS: what would you do? *BMJ* 2007; **334**: 181.

Chapter 5

Evidence-based medicine and the codification of knowledge

Unhampered by any knowledge of bedside care, many non-clinicians, economists and politicians speak with clarity on a difficult subject
P.B. Fowler (1997)[1]

The process of industrialization requires the formation of a body of knowledge that standardizes practice. Professional bodies have always sought to define good practice, and have always measured applicants for entry against their standards of good practice, but (until recently) they have not sought to control the quality of everyday clinical work. Now scientific knowledge has to be aggregated, analysed by detached experts and shaped into the correct way to work, so that the healthcare industry can always produce the same results, or solve the same problems in more or less the same sort of way. The transition from professional description of best practice to systematic external prescription of good quality clinical care is a defining feature of industrialization.

In medicine professional knowledge has traditionally been set out in textbooks that summarize clinical experience and the findings of research in ways that allow the practitioner to infer best practice in most situations. The electronic versions of the *British National Formulary* or the Short Oxford textbook provide the on-line versions and are the surviving examples of this. More recently professional organizations, voluntary bodies, and the National Health Service (NHS) itself have developed 'guidelines', topic-specific textbooks that condense knowledge succinctly and express best practice explicitly.

The most recent versions of these, stemming from the National Institute for Health & Clinical Excellence (NICE), combine evidence-based approaches to medicine, professional consensus about best quality care and criteria and benchmarks for auditing performance—a combination that is designed to standardize practice. Every time we visit the NICE website for the latest advice, discuss concordance with guidelines with registrars or the practice team, or respond to the Quality Outcomes Framework alerts in the record of the patient sitting across from us, we are enacting the industrialization of general practice. Our understanding and use of, and relationship to, 'evidence', has been transformed in just over a decade, from the time that evidence-based medicine (EBM), a by-product of a North American approach to medical education[2] took the NHS by storm in the 1990s.

EBM became the 'Big Idea' of the NHS in the mid-nineties, and has had a huge impact on continuing medical education, policy-making, and service development, and on the research agenda of the health services. At its most general it can be described as the 'conscientious, explicit and judicious use of robust evidence in making decisions about the care of individual patients'.[3] Some of its founders said, by way of justifying their zealous crusading for EBM: 'We become out of date and our patients pay the price for our obsolescence.'[4] This is unarguable, and as no doctor can object to the idea that medical treatment should be based on the best available evidence, the concept of EBM should not be contentious. Yet its promotion provoked resistance and controversy at the time, as an exchange of correspondence in the *Lancet* demonstrated.[5–8] Norman[7] pointed out the paradox of how EBM was promoted as an essential part of every clinician's thinking and working, in reviewing the study of inpatient care in one work unit where the clinicians' practice was found to be in accordance with published evidence in over 80% of cases. Had this result been typical of clinical practice in hospitals then EBM itself did not need so much promotion, for the traditional method of sifting scientific knowledge and disseminating new findings through local professional authority seemed to be functioning in four of five cases. If, on the other hand, the result was so good because of the presence on the medical team of an EBM expert then only a limited number of such experts would be needed and not all clinicians would need to become acquainted with the techniques of EBM itself. Either way EBM was a tool with some use, but not quite the revolutionary discipline set to transform medicine as its advocates hoped.[7]

The views expressed in the *Lancet* correspondence remain relevant because they show how the advocates of EBM were anything but cautious and tentative in their claims, and how annoyed they became when asked for evidence that their approach actually improved outcomes for patients. Entertaining though the debates were, the hyperbole and tetchiness of the more zealous proponents of EBM are the least of its problems, and it continues to attract criticism from the perspectives of political economy, medical humanism, and scientific methodology. Understanding these criticisms may help us to see how well or badly EBM fits with everyday general practice, and how useful or problematic it may be for industrialized primary care.

The dark side of evidence-based medicine

Mykhalovskiy and Weir summarized the political criticisms of EBM in a perceptive review in *Social Science and Medicine* in 2004.[9] From the viewpoint of political economy, enthusiasm for EBM among clinicians seems naïve, when it is considered in the context of health services dominated (as in the USA) or at least heavily influenced (as in the UK) by market mechanisms and subject to continuous cost-containment policies. Its numerically based aggregated knowledge corrodes medical judgement and makes medical practice controllable, ties doctors' decision-making to financial imperatives, transforms itself easily into business knowledge of pathways and protocols, and legitimizes the withdrawal of services from the public.

The humanist critique attacks the 'heartless application of knowledge to the verdancy of patient experience', arguing that people are reduced to the status of objects and professionals to the roles of technicians. EBM undermines the general practitioner (GP) as a listener and counsellor, and strips her patients of their stories, fragmenting and reifying unique individuals. For example, clinicians and patients judge success by the way in which the ill patient becomes better, which is an individual-specific outcome difficult to measure with the kind of standard scales that randomized controlled trials (RCTs) depend upon.[10] The scientific evidence is drawn from RCTs that bear little relationship to real-life clinical situations, and so lack external validity. The methods for distilling evidence are doctor-centred rather than patient-centred, or, as GP Kevork Hopayian has pointed out,[11] so biased towards the techniques of sifting evidence and judging rigour that they are of limited clinical value. Large numbers of systematic reviews show no effect or insufficient evidence, and there can be a high level of subjective interpretation in reading systematic reviews, with authors being more optimistic in conclusions than readers.[12] The research output that EBM depends upon is therefore insufficient to describe 'best practice'[13] in many clinical scenarios.

Finally, EBM subverts political decisions about healthcare by repackaging them as technical problems to be solved by experts in the analysis of knowledge. It is a form of 'technological oppression', an example of what Foucault called 'negative power' operating through negation, shutting down, and deduction. Its use to justify the rationalization of health services is, therefore, no surprise.

These criticisms have some resonance and power, and it is not surprising that some of EBM's 'early adopters' slipped quietly off the bandwagon as the debates intensified. The rhetoric of purity that surrounded EBM in its early days, the sense that a status claim to holiness was being made, and the assorted conversion narratives of doctors who had seen the light, tarnished the image of EBM for some. However, religious comparisons aside, the criticisms are also challengeable, in part because they are weak on empirical evidence and tend to strip EBM out of its context within the NHS. Mykhalovskiy and Weir go some way to explaining why EBM has colonized the whole of medicine in the UK, and spread into healthcare systems much less centralized than ours.

In defence of evidence-based medicine

The pioneers of EBM were not humble, but their goals were never aligned to budgetary thinking, and from the outset they promoted the connection of secure knowledge to practice through skilled reading of evidence by independent doctors. Such 'clinical epidemiology' might seem to be an oxymoron, but arguably the EBM attempt to resolve the apparent contradiction between population-based evidence and the treatment of individuals could increase professional autonomy, knowledge, and status rather than reduce it. They were also concerned with the inequities that occur when the same problem is managed differently by different doctors, and they never expected knowledge to be monopolized by doctors, making them more democratic than their critics claimed. The actual ways in which EBM is being applied, as in NICE guidelines, does combine finely sifted scientific evidence with professional judgement and lay perspectives, undermining the view that EBM is the triumph of the academic over the practical. And the local application of guidelines relies on flexibility and modification, not closure of judgement, giving EBM 'positive power' because it enables development rather than limits it.

We could dismiss the intentions of EBM's advocates as either irrelevant or hopelessly optimistic, but the accumulating experience of developing and implementing guidelines is less easy to ignore. The collective construction of prescriptions for good practice is an educational experience, at least for guideline writers, which could also facilitate the enrolment of GPs into the soft bureaucracy, and promote the specialization and collaboration needed for forward integration of local services. EBM may be less of a hazard to the biopsychosocial approach of general practice than we might think, even if EBM is sometimes expropriated for rationing purposes, precisely because it emphasizes the role of the critical thinker. There is, however, a further tranche of criticism that may prove more damaging to EBM in the eyes of GPs, and that is the challenge to its scientific robustness.

What is evidence?

David Byrne, Professor of Sociology and Social Policy at Durham University, argues cogently that there is a fundamental problem for those encouraging practitioners to act on evidence when that evidence is drawn almost exclusively from RCTs and other kinds of experiment.[3] These, he states very firmly, provide useful information that paints a picture of populations and so are useful to public health doctors and for service commissioning. The attraction of EBM to NHS managers lies in its capacity to challenge professional influence by disputing what and how doctors know, medical knowledge being seen as inherently and irretrievably uncertain. The pursuit of 'hard', objective, impersonal data is driven by a desire for certainty, and promises definitive solutions that might reduce variations in practice and minimize waste[14]. However, probabilistic explanations of the kind generated by RCTs create a picture of reality that is true over large numbers of instances and over time, but individual events (like any common problem encountered in general practice) are unique and statistically independent, and practitioners cannot know how to respond to them by using probabilistic evidence. Although EBM's approaches, and in particular the preoccupation with outcomes, claim to provide clinicians with more certainty, they only increase our certainty about what is probable, and may even increase the uncertainty of practitioners who have to work out how to apply a badly formulated or ill-fitting guideline recommendation.[15] The temptation to reduce the complexity of clinical practice and consider, for example, only the treatment of a 'primary diagnosis' neglects the problems of caring for patients with multiple pathology, or without diagnoses at all.[6] In addition, the population sampling in mega-trials is non-random and subject to large selection biases, and trials are often conducted in specialized research settings rather than in workaday practice, making the generalizability and applicability of trial results even less powerful.[16]

RCTs, however pragmatic, have a mono-causal explanation of events built into their design while most of the reality that practitioners encounter has events with multiple causes, whether they are acute coronary events or instances of domestic violence. Practitioners are more determinist than probabilistic in thinking, using personal experience and extensive knowledge alongside research evidence, justifying the mix and match approach on the pragmatic ground that it is relevant to the complexities of patients and illnesses.[17] We work in ways that are 'deterministic (that is ... clinical events necessarily have causes that can be identified and ... modified) and realistic or naturalistic (this entails a belief in a world of objectively real entities whose nature can be observed)'.[18] The response to this criticism that EBM includes an interest in getting research into practice[19] is not entirely convincing, given the preoccupation of EBM publications with the critical appraisal of trials and its neglect of the huge cultural and communication gap between research workers and practitioners.[20] Central assumptions of EBM are often not shared by GPs,[21] and the EBM approach influences public health specialists and commissioners more than practitioners,[22] with relatively low uptake of evidence-based guidelines,[23] at least in the early years.

In general practice we work (quite rightly in Byrne's view) through the intensive study of limited number of events or cases, apply a 'science of clues' and develop complex models of causality that are context-specific—in my practice what was true for the health-seeking behaviour of refugees from Kosovo does not necessarily apply to affluent city-dwellers dreaming of escaping to the countryside. This whole process requires theories to emerge through enquiry and be modified by it, whereas RCTs require a theory to be produced first and then tested in a separate process. The scientific limitations of RCTs are so extensive that they simply cannot be used as a gold standard for evidence of what works in practice. Professor Byrne's last thoughts are about the reasons for the intellectual dominance of the RCT in scientific methodology, his conclusion being that trials allow medical scientists to be 'little gods' who tinker with the world. This is an appealing explanation but we will return to this question, because there are other less pejorative answers.

The changes that have occurred in EBM over the last decade suggest that its critics have had an impact. Guidelines now produced by NICE do not rank evidence according a hierarchic schema with RCTs at the pinnacle and professional opinion at the (near worthless) base. Professional judgement is given an important place, as are lay perceptions and opinions, and other forms of evidence—such as observational studies or mathematical modelling—are thrown into the guideline pot and stirred until a final product takes shape. The criteria for choosing a clinical problem for an evidence-based approach are interesting because they include: the degree of uncertainty about best practice (as measured through practice variations), the clinical burden, the amount of evidence on cost-effectiveness, the likelihood of engaging clinicians and changing practice, and the possibility of achieving consensus.[24] The strength of evidence is not in this list, which reflects practice concerns and realities more than scientific ones in a way that GP managers being drawn into the industrialized structure of primary care should note carefully. This shift is an important success for a realist approach to the evaluation of evidence, and endorses the involvement of GPs in guideline development and implementation. The detailed debates on the philosophy of science are not necessarily our core concern, but the complex thinking that goes on in everyday clinical work is coming closer to being rehabilitated as a valid approach to science, and GPs will no doubt continue to contribute to its resurgence.

Why is evidence-based medicine so powerful?

EBM is not the only contender for the 'big idea in medicine' title, but it is at the moment the most prominent, and despite all the qualifications cited above has probably changed medical thinking and to a lesser extent practice more extensively than management or clinical governance. 'Patient-centred' medicine is an alternative concept that few clinicians could resist as it starts from the concrete deontological perspective of doing the best possible for the individual patient now sitting in the consulting room. If it could be promoted as the central tenet of general practice it might further enhance communication skills, foster understanding of the sociology of knowledge, behaviour change, and therapeutic interventions, and set a research agenda that includes gender, race and class as key themes. If it allowed for a Quality Outcomes Framework at all, it would not necessarily collect the same sorts of data in the same ways as the 2004 GP contract. Patient satisfaction might be more prominent (and might be better measured), and satisfactory resolution of complex problems might be another marker, perhaps captured using critical incident techniques applied to perceived successes and failures rather than through remote data extraction from electronic medical records. Sennet's Disc World would give way to 'interpretative modulation' of reports of complex clinical scenarios.

'Community Oriented Primary Care' (COPC) is another, perhaps more contentious, rival idea that would focus on need's assessment and unmet need, barriers to service use, public involvement in priority setting, service development and management, and patient involvement in decision-making about and implementation of treatments. This is a more utilitarian view that emphasizes the best outcomes for the highest priority problems in a community, and has obvious affinities with public health medicine, and connections too with community development methods. This approach contains enough measurable population-level indicators to have a rival Quality Outcomes Framework, but even then the amount of social knowledge needed to implement COPC effectively might prove difficult to capture. Neither of these rivals come close to challenging the pre-eminence of EBM. How did EBM become such an attractive idea? How does it continue to outstrip its rivals? What gave it the power to launch journals, influence health service mangers and invade curricula?

One way to think about this is to treat EBM as its authors intended, as an instrument for change, a new technology to be applied to professional activity and to health service development, and as a multipurpose tool, adaptable to all disciplines. Technology development is an interesting field that has some parallels with genetics[25] allowing us to think about new instruments as hybrids, mutations, recombinants, and metamorphs. As a set of ideas EBM is not just the mixing of old ideas into a new *hybrid*, nor is it a small and narrow *mutation* of ideas. Within EBM ideas about the practice of scientific medicine have been reshuffled to make a product that is much more powerful than the sum of its parts—a *recombinant*. The advocates of EBM may want it to be a *metamorph*, producing a dramatic and visible change in the next generation of clinicians.

Much of the argument around EBM is about its rightful character, as evolutionary recombinant or as revolutionary metamorph, and the early debates gave us good insight into the actual contribution that EBM might make to clinical practice (as opposed to the rhetorical claims). Reducing the complexity of practice leads to only a limited range of treatment outcomes for patients being considered, largely those that are easily quantified. In the example given by Rosenberg and Donald in the *British Medical Journal* in 1995[19] of an older woman with non-rheumatic asymptomatic atrial fibrillation, the EBM approach recommends lifelong warfarin treatment because randomized trials show a reduced risk of stroke following this course. Three other important outcomes were not included in the risk–benefit analysis,[26] presumably because they were harder to quantify and had not yet been studied in trials. They were the costs to the patient and to the healthcare system of daily treatment and regular monitoring; the potential disruption to current or future drug treatments for other conditions; and the results of imposing the sick role by treatment of an asymptomatic condition.

In response to such criticism advocates of EBM argued that they did not seek to impose a 'party line' on clinical practice and that the circumstances of the patient will determine *actual* treatment.[8,27] Rosenberg and Donald[19] demonstrate this qualification of EBM's rigour in their example of the treatment of atrial fibrillation by choosing an INR range at the lower end of that shown by trials to be effective because they believe this to be 'safer for the patient'. Their approach was sensible, but deflates EBM's profile somewhat and makes it into a rather limited way of making a bit more sense of the problems clinicians face. The qualifications to the power of their approach that the proponents of EBM must introduce when challenged make their methods more of a recombinant (a useful tool) and less like a metamorph (a discipline in its own right). When the patient's perspective is included in the debate, the position of EBM as arbiter of correct clinical judgement or prudent service provision is further weakened. Some patients may opt for treatments that have been shown to be less efficacious than others by EBM, and purchasers may agree to fund such treatments, because patient choice may reflect a complex comparison of benefits and risks, different weightings of severities of outcome and different valuations of time that do not correspond to the EBM view.[28]

Attacker's advantage?

This argument is important, but the future of EBM does not depend on the outcome of academic debates, but on the outcome of competition with other ideas and on the extent of natural resistance to change found among clinicians. Whether recombinant or metamorph, the success of EBM has depended on its 'attacker's advantage'.[29] Attacker's advantage means the ability either to provide a solution to old problems in a limited but still important market (as a substitution technology), or to extend an existing market (as a replacement technology), or to create a new market for itself (as a placement technology). In my view EBM has become powerful because it appears to function in all three ways.

It is a *substitution technology* because it replaces one method of learning with a cleaner, 'truer' method, in the same way that unleaded petrol has replaced leaded petrol. The market of clinicians remains limited, despite its historic growth, but EBM offers it an educational mechanism based on a structured and systematized scientific method of analysing knowledge itself, and leads away from educational approaches that may be commercially biased (by the pharmaceutical industry), dominated by specialist knowledge (through the teaching hospitals and the traditional research community), or shallow (based on anecdote and case series). Rival ideas such as patient-centred medicine and COPC do not provide a streamlined and more advantageous way of working, possibly because they require very significant changes in power relationships between clinicians and individual patients, or whole communities. EBM has the advantage of keeping scientific developments within the scientific community, even if it does empower researchers more than practitioners.[17] There are potential disadvantages for patients, of course, as scientists determine research objectives, interpret data and may disregard patients' priorities. Ethical standards are determined by powerful groups that define 'gold standard' knowledge and filter out 'inferior' knowledge.[30] All of this reinforces the politically-driven need for public and patient involvement in the development of research itself, as well as in monitoring and shaping practice.

It is also a *replacement technology* because it extends the market for useable scientific knowledge to at least two important groups in medical care, public health physicians and managers. Public health physicians have, through EBM, a policy tool for guiding decisions about purchasing clinical care, just at a time when cost-containment pressures demand the rationing of such care. Before EBM public health doctors who were trained to think epidemiologically had few ways of deciding how to advise on contracts for say, the management of back pain or menorrhagia, and the crisis of identity for public health physicians in a market environment was palpable.

Similarly, managers of health services have in EBM a management tool for controlling clinical activity, something that they have long wanted but never really had. EBM has the potential to further define and improve the quality of care, and to identify 'inappropriate' care and reduce inter-practice variation[24] making it very attractive to managers looking for ways to lubricate performance management. By its assumptions about uncertainty and its almost exclusive reliance on statistical inference, EBM is more conservative than the traditional, deterministic way of medical thinking,[31] prompting the angry response that it is 'a built-in method for rejecting or delaying medical advances'.[1] It is not surprising, therefore, that managed care systems in the USA were early adopters of EBM approaches and guidelines.[32] However, variations in quality of care did not decrease,[33] at least in the initial period of guideline implementation, when we might expect EBM to have had a significant impact. EBM may have less of a real role as a replacement technology than its advocates think. However, it does cement the working relationship between strategic thinking (epitomized by public health medicine) and day-to-day tactical management in ways that patient-centred medicine and COPC could not. To keep all this in perspective we need to remember that decision-making at primary care trust level and above depends on financial constraints, shifting time-scales and experiential knowledge more than research findings, which tend to influence policy debates and mediate dialogue between service providers and users,[34] rather than alter practice.

Finally, EBM is a *placement technology* that creates an entirely new market for ways of understanding medical knowledge, and these will undoubtedly influence practice positively in some areas,[35] as applying an EBM approach improves the quality of medical reasoning.[36] Through practising EBM clinicians will ask more searching questions and obtain more useful answers to them, becoming practitioners in the philosophy of science as well as in its application. To do this they will need teachers and training, books, websites and courses, journals and seminars, and of course, examinations. All these needs will be met by new kinds of educators and scientists, whose expertise will become essential to the proper functioning of medical services in the same way that health economists have become ubiquitous.

To return to the religious analogy cited earlier, a new priesthood will form to create and interpret this new body of knowledge.

EBM appears to have considerable 'attacker's advantage', if only by being different things to different interest groups, and so seems likely to triumph over rival approaches to the codification of knowledge in general practice. It will not do so unmodified, however, because of its fundamental limitations and its sheer instrumentality. It has the potential to create 'additional clinical work around a false standard of clinical certainty',[17] thus generating the very waste its manager advocates thought it might abolish. We have already seen how the production of guidelines is being modified, and we can read with satisfaction that guidelines that have impeccable scientific and methodological pedigrees do not change practice, which remains contingent upon the beliefs and attitudes of professionals, the circumstances in which local organizations find themselves and the priorities and commitments of the NHS.[24] So, if EBM does not lead directly to the unfettered management of clinical knowledge, what other methods can be used to bind practitioners more closely to the aims and objectives of an industrializing health service? The next aspect of industrialization to consider is the modernizing ideology that will allow practitioners to become self-managing within a set of rules laid down from outside: clinical governance.

References

1. Fowler P. Evidence based everything. *J Eval Clin Pract* 1997; **3**(3): 239–43.
2. Sacket DL, Harness RBI, Tugwell P. *Clinical epidemiology: a basic science for clinical medicine*. Boston: Little & Brown, 1985.
3. Byrne D. Evidence-based: What constitutes valid evidence? In *Governing medicine: theory, practice*. Gray A, Harrison S (eds). Open University Press, 2004. pp. 81–92.
4. Sackett D, Richardson W, Scott, Rosenberg, William, Haynes R. *Evidence based medicine: how to practice and teach EBM*. New York: Churchill Livingstone, 1997.
5. Editorial. Evidence based medicine, in its place. *Lancet* 1995; **346**: 785.
6. Bradley F, Field J. Letter. *Lancet* 1995; **346**: 838–9.
7. Norman G Evidence based medicine. *Lancet* 1995; **346**: 839.
8. Sacket D. Evidence based medicine. *Lancet* 1995; **346**: 840.
9. Mykhalovskiy E, Weir L. The problem of evidence-based medicine: directions for social science. *Soc Sci Med* 2004; **59**: 1059–69.

10. Wright G. Evaluating the outcome of treatment: shouldn't we be asking patients if they are better? *J Clin Epidemiol* 2000; **53**(6): 549–53.

11. Hopayian K. The need for caution in interpreting high quality systematic reviews. *BMJ* 2001; **323**: 681–4.

12. Ezzo J, Bausall B, Moerman DE, Berman B, Hadhazy V. How strong is the evidence? How clear are the conclusions? *Int J Health Tech Assessin Health Care* 2001; **17** (4): 457–66.

13. Perleth M, Jakubowski E, Busse R. What is best practice in health care? *Health Policy* 2001; **56**(3): 235–50.

14. Tannenbaum S. Evidence and expertise: the challenge of the outcomes movement to medical professionalism. *Academic Med* 1999; **74**(12): 1259–60.

15. Tannenbaum S. Getting there from here: evidentiary quandaries of the US outcomes movement. *J Eval Clin Pract* 1995; **1**(2): 97–103.

16. Charlton BG. Megatrials are subordinate to medical science. *BMJ* 1995; **311**: 257.

17. Tannenbaum S. Knowing and acting in medical practice: the epistemological politics of outcomes research. *J Health Polit Policy Law* 1994; **19**: 27–44.

18. Harrison S. The politics of evidence based medicine in the United Kingdom. *Policy Polit* 1998; **26**: 15–31.

19. Rosenberg W, Donald A. Evidence based medicine: an approach to clinical problem solving. *BMJ* 1995; **310**: 1122–6.

20. Owen P. Clinical practice, medical research: bridging the divide between the two cultures. *Br J Gen Pract* 1995; **45**: 557–60.

21. Tomlin Z, Humphrey C, Rogers S. General practitioners' perceptions of effective health care. *BMJ* 1999; **318**(7197): 1532–5.

22. Coleman P, Nicholl J. Influence of evidence-based guidance on health policy and clinical practice in England. *Qual Health Care* 2001; **10**(4): 229–37.

23. Coiera E. Maximising the uptake of evidence into clinical practice: an information economics approach. *Med J Aust* 2001; **174**(9): 467–70.

24. Niessen L, Grijseels E, Rutten F. The evidence based approach in health policy and health care delivery. *Soc Sci Med* 2000; **51**: 859–69.

25. Farrell C. Survival of the fittest technologies. *New Sci* 1993; **137**(1859): 35–9.

26. Smith BH. Quality cannot always be quantified. *BMJ* 1995; **311**: 258.

27. Rosenberg W, Donald A. Authors' reply. *BMJ* 1995; **311**: 259.

28. Jones GW, Sagar SM. No guidance is provided for situations for which evidence is lacking. *BMJ* 1995; **311**: 258.

29. Foster R. *Innovation: the attacker's advantage*. Macmillan Basingstoke 1986.

30. Leeder SR, Rychetnik L. Ethics and evidence-based medicine. *Med J Aust* 2001; **175**(3): 164–7.

31. Keaney M. Proletarianising the professionals: the populist assault on discretionary autonomy. In *The social economics of health care*. Davis J (ed.). London: Routledge, 2001.

32. Shortell S, Zazzali J, Burns L, Alexander J, Gillies R, Budetti P, Waters T, Zuckerman H. Implementing evidence-based med icine—the role of market pressures, compensation incentives and culture in physician organisations. *Med Care* 2001; **39**(7): 162–78.

33. Gross P, Greenfield S, Cretyin S, Ferguson J, Grimshaw J, Grol R, Klazinga N, Lorenz W, Meyer G, Riccobono C, Schoenbaum S, Schyve P, Shaw C. Optimal methjods for guideline implementation—conclusions from the Leeds Castle meeting. *Med Care* 2001; **39**(8): 1185–92.

34. Elliott H, Popay J. How are the policy-makers using evidence? Models of research utilisation and local NHS policy-making. *J Epidemiol Community Health* 2000; **54**(6): 461–8.

35. Walder B, Tramer MR. Evidence-based medicine, systematic reviews in peri-operative medicine—fad or necessity? *Anaethetists* 2001; **50**(9): 689–94.

36. Bornstein B H, Emler AC. Rationality in medical decision making: a review of the literature on doctors' decision-making biases. *J Eval Clin Pract* 2001; **7**(2): 97–107.

Chapter 6

The arrival of clinical governance

We aspire to a world in which patients are
protected by measures of competence; failing
teams and organizations can be identified and
remedial action taken; patients and their
advisers, especially family doctors, can make
informed choices of services to use; and service
commissioners can deploy resources most
efficiently to achieve best care. Finally, the
Treasury can monitor improvements in care and
be held to account by the electorate. This world
is currently far from reality.
Mike Pringle et al. BMJ *(2002)*[1]

The big problem for the managers of the national health service
(NHS) during the early phases of the industrialization of general
practice has been to find ways to synchronize the production and
application of knowledge, to combine soft coercion with the maintenance of trust, and to increase efficiency in the use of resources.[2]
Developing organization-wide systems in primary care teams is difficult,
given the tradition of autonomous decision-making, the lack of experience of whole systems approaches in primary care, and the uni-professional paradigms driving educational policy and practice.[3] Early
attempts in the industrialization process to change the way in which
general practitioners (GPs; and other NHS professionals) worked
were unsuccessful and did not have much impact on the values,
beliefs, and organizational subcultures that underpin practice.[4]

Fundholders, for example, did little to kick-start the retail market desired by the government of the day, and instead maintained as much stability in local health service provision as they could while making small changes to the provision of particular services, such as physiotherapy. Probably the one big change that fundholding engineered was the expansion of practice management itself. Centralized control of clinical practice, through the 1990 contract, prompted changes that appeared to be superficial.

It was obvious by the mid-1990s that the modernization of a fragmented health service into a cohesive industrial whole could not occur through the use of crude mechanisms of market opportunities and imposed contracts, and this awareness prompted the emergence of the much more complex package of levers, incentives, and controls that constitute 'clinical governance'. Clinical governance is an ideology designed to promote the centralized regulation of medicine while simultaneously encouraging 'bottom-up' change in the ways services are delivered. As such, clinical governance could 'inspire and enthuse', when seen from above,[5] but has been less well-received by those who provide clinical services. The contradictoriness of this ideology, both conceptually and in practice, was obvious from the beginning, and generated the charges of 'Stalinism' used or hinted at by the eminent academics quoted at the beginning of this book. Their comparison was with democratic centralism, the mechanism by which democratic debate hardens into a binding resolve within organizations established to overthrow the existing order, and with its consequence, a centralized or guided democracy in which all could freely discuss how they would fulfil the centrally decided plan. Like all ideologies, it is open to interpretation, and where suitably vague in its formulation, to modification. Liam Donaldson and Muir Gray, from their elevated position within the power structure of the NHS, can describe it as 'the means by which the clinical professions can maintain the positive liberty they have enjoyed for so long without, until recently, serious challenge'.[6] A non-clinical academic observing clinical governance from outside the NHS can argue that 'clinical governance entails a variety of mechanisms aimed at securing greater managerial control of ... medicine ... a shift from governance based on "communion" to governance based on "command"'.[7]

Like evidence-based medicine, clinical governance is different things to different people, only more so. Here are some of the things that different authors think clinical governance includes:

- Balancing clinical autonomy and professional self-determination with a sense of collective responsibility, in a reformulation of the public good as it applies to general practice.[8]

- 'Selling' changes in behaviour to diverse and disparate professional groups and interests.[8]

- Establishing dialogue to promote collective thinking and 'whole systems working'.[9]

- Assuring quality in existing services and improving the future quality of care,[10] and living with the conflict between the two (between monitoring today's practice and nurturing tomorrow's).

- Fostering accountability downwards to patients and communities, sideways to peers and upwards to the management structure of the NHS,[11] while accepting that in periods of resource constraint only the latter will have priority.

This collection of tasks requires a number of ingredients for success, including:[8]

- Strong medical leadership.

- The continued input of the new breed of practice managers that emerged during the first phase of industrialization.

- Support for those leading change, who are vulnerable in 'the emotionally charged climate in which clinical governance is being established.'

- Clarity about what clinical governance is and includes, being more than audit but less than a complete system of quality assurance.

The more the attributes stack up, the more clinical governance begins to look like the political thinking and activity of a changing public domain, in which GPs are drawing closer to becoming members of the public sector. Most writers on clinical governance see the emergence of this political culture in problematic terms. They identify three types of problem: (1) the difficulty of promoting worthwhile change in general practice, for a variety of reasons; (2) the likelihood of a change of direction in clinical governance that could undo the small changes achieved to date; and (3) the need for substantial support and resources.

Promoting change

The very diversity of general practice makes the development of a political culture of clinical governance that seeks, among other objectives, the standardization of primary care very difficult to achieve.[8] The move away from uni-disciplinary education to multidisciplinary team based learning that seems central to clinical governance requires a number of obstacles to be overcome, not the smallest being our lack of knowledge of how to do it.[12] Limited resources and a slow pace of change may mean that improvements in the quality of care become elusive,[13] while extending the accountability of GPs may generate unsustainable tensions and destructive conflicts. Accountability includes demonstrable fiscal probity, process accountability (having 'proper' procedures such as CHD registers), programme accountability (providing quality care and being concordant with guidelines), and showing that work priorities are relevant or appropriate.[11] This is a big enough list of tasks, when applied to a service that spans childbirth to death and that has thousands of work units, but it becomes frighteningly large when the directions of accountability are included. The image in Figure 6.1, modified from Pauline Allen's *British Medical Journal* review,[11] is revealing.

Three things stand out from this figure. First, the arrows of accountability are uni-directional (as they were in the original image). There is no sense that the NHS hierarchy is accountable to GPs or to local communities, or that patients are accountable to anyone. There is no logical reason why the lines of accountability have to be so uniformly uni-directional, and we shall see later in this chapter that an alternative set of relationships is possible. The second is that even this pattern of accountability may represents a shift back towards what Marquand described as an earlier form of professionalism, in which doctors are professional because they act in the public interest rather than because they have special expertise, and therefore fits well with the inherently anti-market character of general practice. While the development of clinical governance as a new political culture of the public domain may be slow, it may not be swimming against the tide,

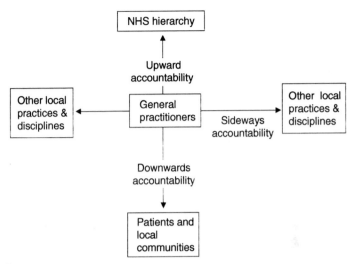

Fig. 6.1

but with it. The third is that, if the lines are seen as representing centrifugal forces, the people in the middle will have an uncomfortable time, particularly when 'the views of the public may not coincide with the goals of the centrally managed NHS'.[11] In a sense GPs have always been pulled between the needs or demands of their patients and the requirements or limitations of either the NHS apparatus or hospital services. Traditionally we have had to mediate between the obvious need for counselling services and the refusal of Family Practitioner Committees or later equivalents to permit the creative use of staff funding for such therapy. We have also become patient advocates by default when ill people endure intolerably long waits for outpatient appointments, elective surgery, imaging, or remedial therapies. Clinical governance may add to these experiences by fostering some sense of accountability to local peers, but there is at least some prospect that a locally collective approach could alter the way services perform, through practice-based commissioning.

Rebalancing clinical governance

The more we explore the ideas wrapped up in the notion of clinical governance, the more they seem appropriate for the continued development of general practice. Even if the financial strings attached to mass production medicine did not influence practices, there would still be merit in cautiously testing out clinical governance as a guide to development. Caution is necessary because the ideas are sometimes vague and the obstacles to making rapid progress are numerous. Among those obstacles is the possibility that the NHS may change its approach to clinical governance, particularly if a new government becomes less interested in investment in public services. So far Primary Care Trusts (PCTs) establishing the structures for clinical governance—the clinical leads, the committees, the procedures—have tended to emphasize their developmental role in achieving future quality rather than their immediate task of monitoring current practice,[10] probably because their leaderships understand the need for conflict avoidance. Sanctions and disciplinary action were not used much, at least initially, and disciplinary roles were transferred upwards to health authorities.[13] This could easily change, especially because tensions between downwards and upwards accountability, in a context of resource limitations, are likely to ensure that upwards accountability is given first priority.[11] We saw in Chapter 4 how monitoring of clinical activity is being mechanized and automated, bypassing the modulating functions of the PCT, and in Chapter 7 we shall see how poorly equipped the NHS is to promote and maintain downward accountability. The balance between soft coercion and the maintenance of trust may shift towards the harder end, provoking conflicts between NHS management and GPs, and potentially between GP managers and their clinical constituencies, as political imperatives to deliver rapid change leads managers to adopt an increasingly authoritarian style.[14]

The need for support

The tasks of clinical governance do seem complex and demanding, and the case for supporting the emerging cadre of primary care leaders made by Mike Pringle,[12] with adequately funded infrastructures,[13] seems convincing. Practitioners learning and applying the new political ideology of clinical governance will need time out of patient contact for training, intelligence-gathering in their local professional communities, reflection, negotiation, and the education of others. They will need training materials and courses, mentoring, and opportunities to exchange views and experiences with their political peer group. The hours spent on this immaterial labour will be paid at the same rate as clinical work, as if they were of equal value, and all the activities that underpin their work will need organizing by secretaries and administrators who are not organizing patient care.

There are two reasons to doubt that all this resource-intensive effort is really necessary. The first is that most practices acquiesced to clinical governance early in the second phase of industrialization, even if they did not embrace it with enthusiasm. If we accept Rudolph Klein's view of the financial orientation of GPs, the prosperity brought to general practice by the 2004 new General Medical Services (GMS) contract will have encouraged even more acquiescence. Other disciplines have absorbed the ideas of clinical governance with seeming ease. Brian Brown and Paul Crawford, in a study of a community mental health team published in *Social Science and Medicine*,[15] describe how 'management is increasingly located inside the individual practitioner' in a form of 'clinical governance of the soul'. Their observation of the way in which CMHT members worked together led them to the conclusions that 'management can work most effectively even when it appears to be invisible or ineffectual' and that 'Professionals who are simply "left to get on with it" have, in a sense, been managed most effectively because they have absorbed sufficient of the ... ideology to construct a way of driving themselves on with the task.' This internalization of clinical governance even thrives on opposition, because the 'autonomous, productive subjectivity of the enterprising professional has become an ever more central resource in the health service.' As we saw with the case of the Derbyshire PCT, those who say 'to hell with the market' are those most needed for the industrialization of general practice into primary care.

The second is that the qualities associated with improving the quality of clinical practice are known:[16] personal involvement in audit, good team working, recognition of the need for a systematic approach to quality improvement, and commitment to continued monitoring of care. These are mostly professional attitudes and ways of working, needing experience and the application of simple principles in practice rather than expensive support and infrastructure. This perspective on improving the quality of services is promoted by the NHS as a 'lean' approach that allows practitioners to work smarter without working harder,[17] and without absorbing extra resources. Lean thinking about clinical governance would look at the well-developed networks of trainers' workshops with their focus on learning environments, the deaneries and their infrastructure, and the practice development awards of the Royal College of General Practitioners and see in them and their successes the necessary and sufficient basis for further changing the political culture of general practice.

Opportunities for general practice

Clinical governance, then, can be seen as a political ideology of the public domain that depends on the engagement of the most positive attributes of GPs—our autonomy and our fund of local knowledge (however partial)—to enhance the quality of care. It can be absorbed and implemented by GPs, practice nurses, psychologists, and counsellors as well as practice managers, if given enough time, and quite possibly only limited extra resources. Its emphasis on professionalism as doing public good—enhancing the quality of clinical care, being accountable in several directions—is in opposition to the definition of professionalism as having special expertise. This latter view is best fitted to the market-place, which is a problem for general practice because our marketable qualities, such as 'holistic' care and the management of uncertainty, are weak attributes compared with the narrower technical expertise of specialists, and lack attacker's advantage. The models of clinical governance currently on offer are simplistic, particularly those of accountability, and are vulnerable to being highjacked by political centralizers within the State, but they are also malleable. The health and illnesses of populations are complex issues that cannot easily be reduced to simple models, forcing us to think about more complex ways of describing the tasks of primary care. These are important issues for general practice that seem worth exploring further, particular in understanding how medical knowledge is actually made and applied in primary care, and how different methods of governance can function. There are also different ways of understanding the embeddedness of general practice within medical science, financial and legal systems, social structures, and community pressures, which means that there are also different ways of shaping clinical governance as a political culture of the public domain.

Medical knowledge

The industrialization of general practice into primary care depends upon a particular way of thinking about how medical knowledge is applied to the problems that people bring to their doctors. This way of thinking is scientific, in that it promises a secure body of knowledge (evidence-based medicine) that can be used for rational decision-making about clinical situations, but it is also structured in ways that allow actual clinical activity to be observed and compared with an ideal model of clinical activity, by people who are not necessarily clinically experienced. It is a way of thinking that shapes medical knowledge for managers as much as for practitioners, and so can be described as 'bureaucratic' as well as scientific.[18]

As we have seen from the discussion of evidence-based medicine, the codification of knowledge in forms amenable to managing clinical encounters from both practitioner and system-organizer perspectives, relies on a series of assumptions about what medical knowledge is and how it can be, or should be, put into practice.[19] The first assumption is that research generates reliable and valid knowledge, and so underlines the importance of academic medicine in finding out the 'truth' about illnesses and diseases, and the effectiveness of treatments and therapies. The second assumption is that practitioners will not be able to sift through the evidence generated by research, so another group of academics will be needed to synthesize the evidence and turn it into practical rules, tools, and guidelines. The third assumption is that the rules describe a logical path through the body of knowledge, allowing practitioners to solve problems in a step-wise fashion, a bit like assembling flat-pack furniture or making a model aeroplane, but not like making a jigsaw.

These assumptions are attractive, and create a hierarchy of knowledge management that is attractive to academia because it not only gives it privileged status over practice, but also channels resources into universities to expand research programmes and to synthesize the knowledge that they generate. It is hardly surprising, then, that clinical governance has emerged through the alliance of managerial and academic interests, as a solution to the problems of providing an expanding repertoire of medical care to increasingly knowledgeable and expectant populations. The problem for those promoting the industrialization of general practice, however, is that the assumptions are insufficient to explain what goes on in everyday clinical work in the community, which is messy rather than linear, complex rather than simple and reliant on knowledge that is not founded on the results of randomized controlled trials (if only because the research evidence base is far smaller than the range of problems encountered).

It is not that we do not like linearity in decision-making, it is that we have too few opportunities to use it because the patients that we see are often too complex for simple algorithms to apply to them, or the algorithms do not yet exist in a reliable enough form. Just think how much heart-rise there is an antenatal care, where a step-wise rule system can be applied to a situation which may not be problematic at all, and compare that with the unpicking of the complaint of 'dizziness' or of being 'tired all the time'. Meeting a patient with only a sore throat is different entirely from the worried but probably well individual with a list of disparate complaints and symptoms. In practice we have little choice but to rely on tacit reasoning—the hidden, problem-solving logic that has developed through experience—and the rules of thumb (heuristics) that we derive from it. This reasoning may become less tacit if we have the opportunity to discuss the clinical problem with others, so that decision-making may be altered by debate, negotiation, and revision, but even then the absence or skimpiness of scientific evidence forces creativity on collective thinking.

The reality of clinical work in general practice is that it is very often iterative rather than linear, exploratory rather than decisive, and episodic rather than continuous. Jan de Lepeleire's accounts of how GPs think around and about the problem of failing memory and reasoning in older patients in complex, often repetitive ways over time are welcome antidotes to the step-wise reasoning of the clinical algorithm.[20] The symptom of memory loss has many possible explanations and implications, and its meaning will depend upon who reports it, who is affected by it, what medical, social, or psychological realities underlie it, and the consequences might be if the symptom of memory loss is connected to its (possibly several) causes in the process of diagnosis. Getting the diagnostic process wrong may have serious effects on everyday life for the person concerned, either because a manageable condition is 'missed', or because false certainty precipitates the person concerned into anxiety, depression, and the risk of becoming socially disabled by the stigma of disease. Not surprisingly GPs check their facts, hypotheses, and hunches many times in exploring memory loss, circling the problem to look at it in different ways, before committing themselves to a diagnosis.

There are two problems here for the development of clinical governance. If clinical governance requires selling changes in behaviour to somewhat sceptical practitioners and establishing dialogue with them to promote collective thinking and 'whole systems working', its proponents will need to work with the grain of clinical reasoning in general practice (the science of clues), not against it. This is likely to mean that changes will begin slowly, even if they then accelerate, and this may not fit with the plans of the PCT or the NHS leadership. The second problem is that our tacit knowledge can make expert knowledge—of the kind privileged by the current thinking about clinical governance—almost redundant, while filtering evidence in conservative ways that protect our own beliefs. By emphasizing the complexity of clinical realities, the paucity of the evidence and the need for experience-based knowledge, we can become a powerful force for stasis in the development of knowledge and practice. The culture of clinical practice then resists change, and becomes the target for managers required to industrialize the whole process of clinical care. One way in which they attempt to overcome this resistance is to emphasize their own (linear) rationality as the only possible rationality, and then to characterize those who resist it as irrational.[21] The climate in which clinical governance is being established could indeed become 'emotionally charged'.

Forms of governance

Faced with resistance to change among practitioners who provide the front-line care in the health service, managers pursuing the industrialization agenda have to use a variety of methods for asserting their superior rationality. This mix and match approach to governance in general practice has three forms, which coexist in different patterns in different situations:[22]

1. Command governance, a hierarchical control of activity, driven by rules.
2. Communion governance, with shared values and frames of reference, and professional leadership.
3. Contract governance, with inducement-contribution exchange.

The reforms of primary care that occurred in the second phase of industrialization, around the 2004 new GMS contract, are a good example of the coexistence of all three methods of including professionals in the industrialization of the whole system. Centrally-driven targets and objectives are being use to shift organizational relationships on to a market basis (command governance), professional bodies are being engaged in the ratification or promotion of such change (communion governance), and remuneration systems are modified to include incentives to become concordant with highly focused clinical objectives (contract governance). Through this mixture of approaches clinical autonomy becomes regulated, managerial strategies are oriented to promoting political centralization, and flexibility and decentralization coexist with rigid structures of domination in the system of 'soft bureaucracy'[23] that we discussed in Chapter 2. Such a 'mix and match' approach sounds as if it might be flexible and sensitive to both patient and professional need, but this is not necessarily the case.

The controversy about the Measles, Mumps & Rubella (MMR) vaccine is a case study of clinical governance and its effects on trust between patients and professionals, and between professionals of different disciplines.[24] Setting targets for MMR immunization makes sense because it combines a managerial objective with a clinical one of maintaining 'herd immunity'. Before a *Lancet* publication suggesting a link between autism and MMR immunization those relatively few parents who were not compliant with the immunization schedule could be categorized as chaotic, apathetic, poor, or lazy without great harm to the achievement of targets and to the maintenance of a coherent professional view of the situation. Once the rumour of a link between MMR immunization and autism took hold, the larger number of MMR refuseniks became problematic, and labelling them as 'precious' or prone to have 'bees in the bonnet' was no help. Chasing the MMR target was experienced by some parents as coercive, and perceived as a potential moral hazard because practitioners had a financial interest that might influence their clinical concern to immunize children against serious diseases. Health visitors felt pressured into delivering targets for GPs, just as GPs felt pressured by managers, and any dissent from the Department of Health arguments about MMR were experienced as stepping out of line. While the behaviour of parents, practitioners, and the Department of Health is likely to change over time, mitigating the negative impact of the MMR scare on both child health and trust between providers and users of services, there seems little doubt that 'clinical governance' in the MMR controversy was very much about controlling practice, and very little about incorporating clinical experience and perspectives into policy making and implementation. I will return to the MMR scare as an issue, and its implications for future relationships between citizens and professionals, in the chapter on consumerism.

Changes at practice level

How will we accommodate to the conflicting pressures to change our organization and everyday clinical work, to align ourselves in the spirit of clinical governance? One perspective that attempts to combine managerial and clinical approaches in improving the quality of care provides a detailed specification of how clinical governance could affect a practice, creating a 'new professionalism' in general practice[25]. The key features are:

- ◆ A management and organizational framework for clinical quality improvement.
- ◆ A 'duty of quality' that falls on the practice, not just its members.
- ◆ A comprehensive strategy to improve quality, using tools like audit, risk assessment, and professional development.
- ◆ A named individual charged with leading the processes of change that will improve care.

- A focus on clinical leadership, but with greater external accountability.
- Attention to clinical decision-making, appropriateness, clinical effectiveness, and evidence-based care.
- All set within national guidelines and standards.

This is an agenda that makes sense, from an organizational point of view, and that brings together largely unchallengeable professional commitments to good quality practice. The commitment to a professional agenda around quality of care will satisfy enough practitioners to make them acquiesce to managerial authority, and that will satisfy the leadership of the NHS. The desirable cultural features of general practice, from a clinical governance perspective,[26] can be inferred from the list of desirable attributes, as in the Table 6.1.

Some of these attributes are now built into the 2004 new GMS contract as performance measures, and others—such as learning from other practices and thinking across interfaces—are subsumed within practice-based commissioning. This is, then, the shape that general practice will take for the foreseeable future, and given the slow pace of change that is necessary to develop such characteristics, we should

Table 6.1

Desirable attribute	Necessary practice characteristic
Accountability	Willingness to demonstrate good quality practice, including publication of comparative data
Learning from other practices	Willingness to learn from others and share experiences and information
User involvement	Focus on partnerships with patients, encouraging greater user participation
Orientation to scientific evidence	Guide clinical practice with scientific evidence
Multiprofessional team working	General practitioners work in partnership with other disciplines
Reflection	Learning constructively from mistakes
Thinking across interfaces	Greater integration of activities across traditional boundaries, such as health and social care or primary and secondary care

probably see it as the agenda for the current new generation entering general practice.

Future proofing general practice

Two things may upset this process of development. The first is a political shift towards more 'command and control' management within the NHS, and the second is the possibility of fierce competition developing between established general practices and new commercial competitors willing and able to invest in buildings and staff, and suffer losses long enough to weaken traditional NHS practices. The consensual approach described above may not then be fit for purpose. Commercial challenges are likely to be localized, and will probably hinge on accessibility and skill-mix rather than governance issues, and we will return to them in the final chapter, but changes in the requirements of centralized management are likely to have a rapid and widespread impact on general practice. If NHS management lurches towards a more authoritarian style then slow change and reflective practice may not offer much protection. Are there alternative ways in which we might shape clinical governance to fit the realities of clinical practice rather better, in ways that could future proof general practice against changes in the political climate?

One alternative approach would be to increase the clinical focus within clinical governance[27] now, by concentrating on:

- The inter-relatedness of clinical practice and resource availability. This may not be politically attractive to government, which wants to show how well it is doing not how constrained it is, nor to PCTs, which may want to deflect attention and criticism away from their rationing decisions by making them as invisible as possible.
- The balance between clinical autonomy and clinical accountability.
- The systematization of clinical work, for example through the development at practice level of case-management methods for care of specific patient groups.
- The devolution of power that needs to occur for team-working to flourish.

Clinical governance in this form would concentrate on describing in detail the content of clinical practice, so that it would be open to self-governance by multidisciplinary teams, but also open to critique by management. The questions that would apply to clinical practice would be about doing the right things, doing things right, meeting all tractable needs for the patient group (or documenting the shortfall) and keeping up-to-date with knowledge.

There may be some lessons on how to do this from outside medicine, particularly from social work, where the complexities are no less than in general practice, the evidence base even thinner and the resource constraints very much worse. Some practical proposals to modifying governance[28] include:

1. Recognizing that 'information' is 'news of difference that makes a difference', and concentrating all efforts to change practitioner behaviour on different ways of working that offer some possibility for solving the practitioners' problems, not just those of the manager.

2. Promoting reflexivity, that is, the discussion of the tacit assumptions that underpin everyday clinical work.

3. Acknowledging that emotional responses to clinical problems or particular patients can influence the way tacit knowledge that is brought to bear in clinical encounters.

4. Assert that the ethics of providing services requires an empathic approach to others, which should be reflected in the process of governance as well as in the content of consultations.

These proposals may have a particular resonance because they are examples of 'immaterial labour',[29] the kind of work that is based on communication, and that encompasses not just problem-solving, analytical thinking, and intellectual abilities, but also emotions and judgements. General practice is immaterial labour in which emotion and judgement take centre stage alongside technical and rational thinking, and GPs balance critical judgements, emotional reactions and reflective thinking in a dynamic way, in every surgery. This expertise may be an advantage for general practice, particularly when practitioners need to review critical incidents and significant events that demand:[30]

1. An understanding of the technicalities of clinical processes.

2. The ability to focus on the systems aspect of errors or failures without lapsing into blame.

3. The capacity to navigate around the emotional politics of investigating the errors of colleagues, friends, or even superiors.

4. Reflection on one's own moral and ethical position.

While there may be consolation for general practice as a discipline in its skilfulness in immaterial labour, compared with specialist disciplines, there are also hazards in this way of working and thinking. GPs could become locked 'into anatomical dissection and publication of its processes, disabling it from intervening in the broader organizational systems and policy processes upon which its practices and risks are contingent.'[30] Committed to good quality clinical care, adaptable as long as clinical autonomy is not usurped, and acquiescent towards the processes of industrialization, GPs may carefully tick the Quality and Outcomes Framework boxes and assiduously fill in the critical incident forms, but neglect the big picture of what is happening to their discipline and the health service.

To acquire a bigger picture we might want with a model of clinical reality that captures more aspects of the real work of general practice than those currently in use in the debates about clinical governance. An example is Engström's model of service development,[31] which identifies macro-level factors influencing clinical practice, and which is particularly useful as a framework for analysing collaborative and co-operative work groups.[32] This model is derived from Activity Theory, which identifies six factors whose interaction facilitates or impedes change:

- The commitment and behaviour of professionals (here taken as doctors and practice nurses).

- The attitudes, expectationsm, and behaviour of patients (here taken as all those registered with the practices).

- 'Instruments'—the knowledge and technology available in primary care.

- The rules governing organization of services, professional conduct, and financing, which subsume local management (the PCTs), national service frameworks, contractual obligations.

- ◆ The 'community', here taken as the local population and the structures of civil society),
- ◆ and division of labour (here taken as both the specialist services available to primary care, and the work distribution in the practices).

This model is represented diagrammatically in Figure 6.2. The bi-directional arrows emphasize the role of relationships in determining change in service provision, without diminishing the importance of the specific content of each of the boxes. The potential importance of the model for us lies in its messiness (which reflects our reality), in the centrality of the doctor–patient relationship and its outcomes, and in the capacity of each component to influence the others, so that the management of the service is responsive to professional or public opinion. Applying the model to a practice or a commissioning group requires the contents of each box to be filled in, and the nature and strengths of the interactions between them to be described. This then makes a unique map of the local services, showing the areas where change in one box could produce or impede changes elsewhere within the system.

Systems thinking

The action theory approach of Engström provides a framework with a high level of generality that permitted us to understand and respond to

Fig. 6.2 Engström's model of service functioning

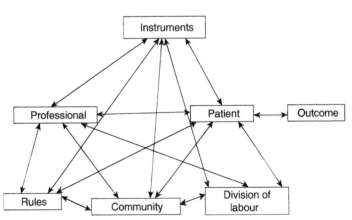

the complexities of individual practices and the heterogeneity of the local practice culture. With it one can appreciate and work with the relationships within practices, and still allow a tailored intervention in practice activity. As a complexity model, this approach allows us to recognize the heterogeneity of organizations and the complex process of translating ideas into actions, in situations where none of the relationships between components of the model could be anticipated accurately. This high-level model permits incorporation of the complexity and richness of relationships between professionals and patients[33] into a wider model of practice organization and work, and offers a whole view of the relationships between multiple components of practice activity, fitting a clinical governance model.[34] In particular it facilitates systems thinking, particularly about the permeability of boundaries[35] and steady states or dynamic equilibria that preserve the system while allowing change and development[36] and the differentiation of systems over time.

The activity theory model allows us to think in terms of non-linear response and feedback loops and so comprehend unanticipated adverse effects, policy resistance, delay, dilution, or the failure of the intervention.[37] The centrality of relationships in the model allows us to include recognition of interpersonal dynamics that can support or prevent change (organizational defence routines),[38] think in terms of causes not symptoms (a diagnostic approach), recognize that leadership skills may matter more than structure or technique, and avoid the pitfalls of 'shared vision' (conformity to prescribed plans, avoidance of reflection) by enabling participants to construct any perspective they wished. Although flexible, the model has definite components prompting analytic discipline, providing sufficient structure to mount an experiment, while avoiding top-down and prescriptive approaches (there is no 'top' and the model is not linear). In my view this model allows interventions at practice level to take account of national policy requirements, local service configurations and other local factors influencing clinical activity, and characteristics of the practices themselves, and should be applicable in any health service that includes family medicine as a discipline. Implementation of an intervention using this model requires policy awareness, local knowledge, and the capacity to read and interpret practice cultures, exactly the attributes required of clinical governance leads.

Implications for education

The approaches to clinical governance discussed in this chapter all have implications for undergraduate and postgraduate medical education, because the current culture of medical training may still be incongruent with the changing nature of general practice, despite the best efforts of the General Medical Council to redefine the core curriculum for medicine and the Deaneries to shape postgraduate training. Undergraduates learn from teachers who adopt the 'sage on the stage' model of the medical role to be 'independent, isolated and competitive' learners who become incisive, confident decision-makers, whose currency is fact-based knowledge'.[39] To function effectively in an environment that is changing in organizational structure, evidence-base and system of funding, graduates need to know how to navigate through complexity and uncertainty on a scale that has not been encountered since the formation of the NHS in 1948. To do this an increasing number of GPs will need to 'question, learn from and understand their own and others' behaviour in teams, how individuals and groups apply factual, personal, and organizational knowledge in different situations, and what would make each group member more able to contribute to knowledge and decision-making.'[40] Postgraduate education in general practice is well developed and one of the greatest assets of the discipline, so we should anticipate a relatively smooth acquisition of clinical governance skills in the rising generation of generalists. The backward diffusion of the clinical governance approach into undergraduate education may be more problematic, but is a fitting task for academic general practice. The most difficult learning, however, will occur as general practice responds to conflicting demands of market-driven medical consumerism and State-sponsored 'producerism', and these are the themes for the next chapter.

References

1. Pringle M, Wilson T, Grol R Measuring 'goodness' in individuals and health-care systems. *BMJ* 2002; **325**: 704–7.
2. Sheaff R, Sibbald B, Campbell S, Roland M, Marshall M, Pickard S, Gask L, Rogers A, Halliwell S. Soft governance and attitudes to clinical quality in English clinical practice. *J Health Serv Res Policy* 2004; **9**(3): 132–8.

3. Evelyn G, Hocking P, Burtonwood A, Harry K, Turner A. learning to plan? A critical fiction about the facilitation of professional and practice development plans in primary care. *J Interprof Care* 2002; **16**(4): 349–58.

4. Nicholls S, Cullen R, O'Neill S, Halligan A. Clinical governance: its origins and foundations. *Br J Clin Governance* 2000; **5**(3): 172–8.

5. Scally G, Donaldson L. Clinical governance and the drive for quality improvement in the new NHS in England. *BMJ* 1998; **317**: 61–5.

6. Donaldson L, Muir Gray J. Clinical governance: a quality duty for health organisations. *Qual Health Care* 1998; 7(Suppl.): S37–44.

7. Harrison S. Governing medicine: governance, science and practice. In *Governing medicine: theory and practice*. Gray A, Harrison S (eds). Maidenhead: Open University Press, 2004, p. 180.

8. Huntington J, Gillam S, Rosen R. Clinical governance in primary care: organisational development for clinical governance. *BMJ* 2000; **321**: 679–82.

9. Pratt J, Gordon P, Plamping D. *Working whole systems: putting theory into practice in organisations*. London: King's Fund, 1999.

10. Campbell S, Sheaff R, Sibbald S, Marshal M, Pickard S, Gask L, Halliwell S, Rogers A, Roland M. Implementing clinical governance in English primary care groups/trusts: reconciling quality improvement and quality assurance. *Qual Saf Health Care* 2002; **11**: 9–14.

11. Allen P. Clinical governance in primary care: accountability for clinical governance: developing responsibility for quality in primary care. *BMJ* 2000; **321**: 608–11.

12. Pringle M. Clinical governance in primary care: participating in clinical governance. *BMJ* 2000; **321**: 737–40.

13. Campbell S, Roland M, Wilkin D. Primary care groups: improving the quality of care through clinical governance. *BMJ* 2001; **322**: 1580–2.

14. Marshall M, Mannion R, Nelson E, Davies H. Managing change in the culture of general practice: qualitative case studies in primary care trusts. *BMJ* 2003; **327**: 599–602.

15. Brown B, Crawford P. The clinical governance of the soul: 'deep management' and the self regulating subject in integrated community mental health teams. *Soc Sci Med* 2003; **56**: 67–81.

16. Stevenson K, Baker R, Farooqi, Sorrie R, Khunti K. Features of primary health care teams associated with successful quality improvement of diabetes care: a qualitative study. *Fam Pract* 2001; **18**: 21–6.

17. *High impact changes for practice teams*. NHS Institute for Innovation & Improvement, 2004.

18. Bilson A, White S. Limits of governance: interrogating the tacit dimensions of clinical practice. In *Governing medicine: theory and practice*. Gray A, Harrison S (eds). Maidenhead: Open University Press, 2004, p. 94.

19. Harrison S. *New Labour, modernisation and health care governance*. London: Political Studies Association/Social Policy Association conference on New Labour, New Health, September 1999.

20. De Lepeleire J, Heyrman J. Diagnosis and management of dementia in primary care at an early stage: the need for a new concept and an adapted procedure. *Theor Med Bioeth* 1999; **20**(3): 215–28.

21. Armstrong JS. Strategies for implementing change: an experimental approach. *Group Organ Stud* 1982; **7**(4): 457–75.

22. Gray A. Governing medicine: an introduction. In *Governing medicine: theory and practice*. Gray A, Harrison S (eds). Maidenhead: Open University Press, 2004, pp. 4–5.

23. Courpasson D. Managerial strategies of domination: power in soft bureaucracies. *Organ Stud* 2000; **21** (1): 141–61.

24. Brownlie J, Howson A. Between the demands of truth and government: health practitioners, trust and immunisation work. *Soc Sci Med* 2005; 2006; **62**: 433–43.

25. Buetow SA, Roland M. Clinical governance: bridging the gap between managerial and clinical approaches to quality of care. *Qual Health Care* 1999; **8**: 184–90.

26. Marshall M, Sheaff R, Rogers A, Campbell S, Halliwell S, Pickard S, Sibbald B, Roland M. A qualitative study of the cultural changes in primary care organisations needed to implement clinical governance. *Br J Gen Pract* 2000; **52**: 641–5.

27. Degeling P, Maxwell S, Iedema R. Restructuring clinical governance to maximise its development potential. In *Governing medicine: theory and practice*. Gray A, Harrison S (eds). Maidenhead: Open University Press, 2004, p. 167.

28. Bilson A, Ross S. *Social work management and practice: systems principles*. London: Jessica Kingsley, 1999.

29. Hardt M, Negri A. *Multitude: war and democracy in the age of Empire*. New York, Penguin, 2004.

30. Iedema R, Jorm C, Long D, Braithwaite J, Travaglia J, Westbrook M. Turning the medical gaze upon itself: root cause analysis and the investigation of clinical error. *Soc Sci Med* 2006; **62**: 1605–15.

31. Engström Y, Miettinen R, Punamä;ki R-L. *Perspectives on activity theory*. Cambridge University Press, 1999.

32. van den Anker F, Bodrozic Z. Activity theory as a basis for analysing co-operative work. In *Dealing with diversity: 5th Congress of the International Society for Cultural Research and Activity Theory, Amsterdam*. van Oers, B, Wardekker W, Blom S, Elber E, Pompert B, van der Veer R (eds). 2002.

33. Neighbour R. *The inner consultation*. Newbury: Petroc Press, 1987.

34. Halligan A, Donaldson L. Implementing clinical governance: turning vision into reality. *BMJ* 2001; **322**: 1413–17.

35. Flood RL. *Rethinking the fifth discipline*. London: Routledge, 1999.

36. Katz D, Kahn RL. *The social psychology of organisations*. New York: Wiley, 1978.

37. Sterman JD. *Business dynamics systems thinking and modelling for a complex world*. Boston, MA: McGraw Hill, 2000.

38. Argyris C. *Overcoming organisational defences, facilitating organisational learning*. Boston, MA: Allyn & Bacon, 1990.

39. Redfern N, Stewart J. What counts is what works: postgraduate medical education and clinical governance. In *Governing medicine: theory and practice*. Gray A, Harrison S (eds). Maidenhead: Open University Press, 2004, p. 140.

40. Redfern N, Stewart J. What counts is what works: postgraduate medical education and clinical governance. In *Governing medicine: theory and practice*. Gray A, Harrison S (eds). Maidenhead: Open University Press, 2004, p. 142.

Chapter 7

What about the patients? Consumerism and producerism in the industrialization process

We are more aware of risks today than our parents were. My mother did not have to make the choices that I am faced with over my family. Everything seems so much harder to deal with today—and it is only going to get more and more difficult as time goes on.

A mother of two small children quoted by Robin McKie & Jo Revill in 'Doctor can't know best', Observer (Sunday 10 August 2003, p. 19)

Seventy percent of the UK population is taking medicines to treat or prevent ill health or to enhance wellbeing. How can this level of medicine taking be appropriate in a population which, by all objective measures, is healthier than ever before in history?

Iona Heath (BMJ April 2005)[1]

It is easy to forget the differences between the individual experience of illness, the social impact of sickness and the pathological processes of diseases. If we forget these distinctions we become confused about why the healthiest and most long-lived populations that have ever existed need so much medical attention. One of the easy answers to this is that providers of medical care generate demand in consumers, and make work for themselves, particularly in economies where this construction of demand is profitable. There is no doubt that this is true, but demand cannot be constructed out of nothing. There has to be some kind of 'want' that the artful seller can manipulate into a 'need' and then 'meet'.

The wants and needs of modern societies are changing, forcing health services built before penicillin was widely available to change their organization and ways of working. There are many dimensions to this social change, from demographic shifts to occupational insecurity, and all of them are having an impact on general practice. They include:

- An ageing population in which multiple medical problems accumulate, requiring prolonged treatment and monitoring.

- The compression of morbidity into a relatively short period at the end of life, a turbulent phase of multisystem failure needing labour-intensive attention from health and social care services.

- The fracturing of value systems in the rising generations that have benefited from the unprecedented freedoms won in the post-war period—freedoms created by the welfare state and the expansion of educational opportunities.

- The unmasking of anxieties, obsessions, and neuroses by increasing affluence, the weakening of self-control and the commercialization of narcissism.

- The formation of a chaotic, unemployable, and unhealthy underclass as the gap between the richest and poorest increases and the market squeezes out those with the least useable skills.

- Ill health promoted by insecurity of unemployment, loss of control over the working environment and a growing sense of injustice.

- Increasing anxieties about risk, in all strata of society.

- Mass migration of populations, for economic and political reasons, from poor and underdeveloped countries into affluent ones, and from war zones to places of relative security.

All of these are already visible in everyday general practice, from the affluent shires to the inner cities, and overlay the dysfunctional coping strategies, personal tragedies, unhappy marriages, collapsing local economies and simple misfortune that filled surgeries throughout the post-war boom, and still occupy our attention. That post-war boom, and its welfare state, permitted the demographic shift, which is now changing the workload of general practice. Increased social mobility and wider access to education, the ability of women to control reproduction and their increasing involvement in the labour market, and the greater leverage that some individuals have over their 'lifestyle' seem to be creating generations that are more autonomous but less trusting than their parents.[2] These generational shifts have been exposed, and perhaps accelerated, by the social change that followed the deregulation of the economy during the Thatcher phase of government. The scale and depth of these changes are sometimes difficult to grasp, because they have been so profound, but we meet their consequences every day. These two trends—the social consequences of prosperity and the effects of commercializing society itself—are already increasing the demands on general practitioners (GPs), and there is no reason to think that this pressure will diminish.

Since 1997 the government has feared that the middle classes would desert the national health service (NHS), effectively turning it into an impoverished safety net service for the poor. Its fear reflects a growing sense of discontent within an articulate and influential minority of the population about medicine broadly and the structures and practices of the health service in particular. This discontent is most visible in younger generations that have little experience of significant illness or disability and no memory of how medical care operated before the NHS, but as we shall see it is by no means confined to them. Those who are becoming the customers of the newly industrialized health service, bring to their dealings with professionals all the lessons learned from encounters across an increasingly commercialized culture. One consequence of this altered relationship is that trust between patients and professionals may be slowly changing from being warm and affect-based to being more critical and cognition-based,[3] making the affability, familiarity and patient-centredness of the GP less important than more obvious signs of competence, knowledgability and skill, plus commitment of time and respect for the patient.

General practice's leaders have tended to respond to this by citing the high levels of satisfaction expressed about GPs, who score 80% on the trustworthiness scale compared with the 20% or less allotted to politicians or journalists. For example, the Department of Health's review of Public Perceptions of the NHS in the Winter of 2004 showed that general practice recorded higher levels of satisfaction (76% satisfied) than any other part of the health service, with little discrepancy between users and non-users of the service, and net satisfaction with the last GP consultation running close to 80%.[4] There is no doubt about the high level of satisfaction when considered in a general sense, but the devil is always in the detail, the definition of the 'public good' is always contested and mutable, and challenges to the routines and customs of professionalism can destabilize the framework of thinking and acting that we take for granted. The seemingly solid fact that four in every five individuals are satisfied overall does not disenfranchise or necessarily disarm the one in five who is disgruntled.

Discontented patients

There are grounds for being concerned at the changes underway in the thinking of citizens about their medical care. In the Healthcare Commission's survey of primary care services in 2004–5[5] just under 117 000 people completed a questionnaire about their experience of general practice. The more educated they were, the more they felt that they had insufficient time to discuss their condition, that they were not treated with respect and dignity, that when referrals were made the information given about them to the specialist was insufficient, and that the specialist (when seen) did not treat them with respect and dignity. Those who rated their health as poor, or who were disabled, were more likely to say that: (1) they had insufficient time in general practice consultations to discuss their condition; (2) they were not involved in care and treatment decisions; (3) explanations were given in terms that they did not understand; and (4) they were not treated with respect and dignity.

We need to think about these associations carefully. Perhaps there is no surprise in the finding that the better educated feel short-changed in the length of consultations, but should we not be concerned at their sense of not being respected? We might expect that the healthy with least contact with the NHS but most exposure to critical media portrayals of medicine would be more prone to a vicarious, almost *ersatz*, dissatisfaction, but the opposite seems to be the case. It is those with the worst health (in their opinion) or those with disabilities who are more dissatisfied, and these are core constituencies of general practice. It may be that those with most experience of general practice are the most likely to be unhappy with their treatment. Older people responded more favourably than younger, perhaps because they compare present experiences with much worse ones in their past, but this may not help us as much as we hope, because positive attitudes to the quality of medical care among older people correlate only weakly with other measures of quality.[6]

This puts us in a difficult position, even if only a minority of our patients are only contemplating the role of the dissatisfied customer. The consumerism that we are now encountering in consultations draws upon the attitudes, values, and techniques of a broader consumerist orientation. It has a traditional component derived from personal experience of the failures of medicine and a new one, born in affluence and linked to the idealization of the rational, autonomous shopper who weighs up the pros and cons of purchases in a market crowded with wares. The traditional consumerist thinking is as reductionist as specialist medicine can be, commodifying health into buyable fragments, but as we shall see the new variant has a much more modern grasp of medical science than the older variant.

The combination of traditional and new forms of consumerism seems likely to make the gatekeeper role of general practice an increasingly conflicted and conflictual one: conflicted because the different explanations and understandings that the modern consumer bring to the doctor–patient relationship will divide professionals, and conflictual because, as consumers, modern patients will want value (as they define it) for the money that they think their taxes represent. We have three different reasons for doubting that this new consumerism will make citizens of the healthiest and longest-living societies in human history into cautious, careful, and considerate users of health services, fully aware of the need to make common use of the common wealth.

First, rationality is not the essence of a consumer society, but a minor, countervailing force against obsessions and compulsions. The emergence of a near-utopia (full employment, increasing free time, rising disposable income) permits the efflorescence of every kind of neurosis and irrationality so that 'no society has ever been quite so addictive, quite so inseparable from the condition of addictiveness as this one, which did not invent gambling ... but which did invent compulsive consumption'.[7] Culture may determine the options for this efflorescence, but binge drinking, widespread recreational drug use and a growing epidemic of cosmetic surgery might dominate the British experience.

Second, the pursuit of wealth by the means advocated by the neo-liberal economists who have dominated North American and British politics since Thatcher and Reagan leads to increased inequality, and the creation of an impoverished and ill underclass that is partially or entirely excluded from usual social life.[8] Richard Wilkinson has shown how stress and insecurity in early life, weak social affiliations and low social status alone or in combination undermine health and promote premature morbidity and mortality.[9] In contemporary Britain a 'carousel effect' pulls poor people back into deprivation just as they struggle to escape it, with precarious, poorly paid employment in a 'flexible' labour market that has a particularly damaging effect on health.[10] We encounter this reality everywhere there are hostels filled with homeless families, in the 'dual diagnosis' of mental illness and drug or alcohol dependency, and the discussions of the child protection case conference. The long-term effects of this poverty within an affluent society on health, the utilization of health services, withdrawal from employment and the uptake of social benefits are clear, for childhood deprivation predicts adult disability.[11]

The gradient of ill health

Widening inequality also has negative effects on the psychological and physical health of those who benefit from the growing affluence, and reduces security, trust, and virtue as money crowds out ethics.[12] The gradient of income produces a gradient of ill-health as multiple stressors challenge the endocrine and immune systems, while the collapse of normal existence may be only a redundancy or one mortgage payment default away. The sense of injustice that develops in this state of insecurity within prosperity is itself hazardous, being associated with a higher risk of coronary heart disease risk even when allowing for age, gender, employment grade, established coronary risk factors and other work-related psychosocial characteristics.[13] At the same time the limits of self-control are overwhelmed by the pervasive insecurity, and novel opportunities for consumption produce tendencies towards seeking short-term rewards, and towards individualism, narcissism, hedonism, and disorientation.[14] The health consequences include, among other trends, the current epidemic of obesity.

Third, a popular consciousness fitted to affluent but competitive societies has a direct effect on the individual's willingness to share the risk of illness with a wider community, and make social provision for sickness and disability. In the North American culture that is now so influential in Europe '… individualistic and narcissistic presuppositions, and, we might say, (socially inscribed) delusions, lead to a systematic under-statement of our dependency on other people in most of our endeavours'.[15] This understates the scale of the problem, because this new consciousness does not describe the body as a collection of parts, but as a complex system with the immune mechanism at its centre, capable of great things but also prone to catastrophic collapse.[16] Just when we think that the basic conditions for a healthy life are available, at least to the affluent, risks increase and catastrophe looms.

Antidotes to consumerism

The state's response to this new, socially malignant consumerism is to try and use it as a way to engineer changes in the way that professionals and the health service work, while also containing its power within a kind of participatory democracy, which acknowledges the potential for individual autonomy in all citizens, but seeks also to incorporate decision-making into a set of relationships and behaviours that are social rather than solitary, reciprocal rather than individualist. The autonomous consumer is rewarded with a Choose and Book approach to outpatient appointments that is modelled on buying airline tickets or package holidays, but in many other aspects of service use consumers are excluded from decision-making and hemmed in by rules about access to services and eligibility for treatments. Participatory democracy is fostered through expert patient programmes and patient surveys that generate results that are interpreted by patient committees. At its extreme this form of public engagement condenses into a form of 'producerism', in which the citizen becomes an idealized co-worker in the production of health.

The attempt to incorporate users of health services into all aspects of medical care, starting with the prioritization and governance of medical research itself and extending across the industry to the choice of hospital, of place of birth and even of the place of death, creates huge tensions within the industry. GPs, by being on the front line of medical care, not only experience the full extent of Adorno's efflorescence of neuroses, but are also required to respond to it while being also urged to engage in the construction of a participatory democracy. This chapter attempts to understand how these tensions affect general practice, as it becomes incorporated into the healthcare industry. First comes consumerism, in its traditional and new forms, and then the public sector's response to it.

Traditional consumerism

Consumerism in medicine combines a buyer's challenge to seller's power with lay resistance to professional authority, and is characterized by doubt and caution (not faith and trust), individual or small group action against professional interests or stances, and the perception of health as a tradeable commodity.[17] This traditional type of medical consumerism probably occurs in all societies and all healthcare systems, and fits within a pattern of conflictual relationships between the citizen and a powerful agency—in our case, the resource allocation role of the GP. Individuals seek their best interests, as they perceive them, by using all the opportunities that the system offers them to gain leverage over decisions, by means of threats ('if I cannot get an appointment I will call a doctor out'), appeals to precedent ('If I don't get antibiotics it always goes to my chest'), or simple bribery (the envelope system in the health services of the former socialist bloc countries literally bought different treatment). Consumer choice can be expressed through seeking alternative opinions in the private sector, or from alternative practitioners.

Consumerism of the traditional kind—shopping around for a preferred diagnosis, treatment, or piece of advice—remains a personal activity, directly related to personal experience.

Traditional consumerist *attitudes* towards medical care appear to be universal, occurring in developed and developing countries, and in market and planned economies. There is nothing new about the scepticism of patients towards doctors, Hippocrates wrote about it. The prescription accepted but not dispensed, the medication not taken, the follow-up appointment made but not kept, may all be features of the doubts and caution that individuals feel about the judgements, opinions, advice, and treatments of their doctors.

Consumerist *behaviour* of the traditional kind, on the other hand, is relatively uncommon except when people are ill. Illness promotes consumerist behaviour when medical care fails to achieve the result desired by the individual. Chronic illness has a particular significance for relationships between citizens and professionals because by definition it cannot be cured by modern medicine. The development of patient behaviour in the course of a chronic illness appears to go through three phases:[18] (1) naïve trust; (2) disenchantment; and (3) guarded alliance. In the beginning the ill individual trusts that the persistent problem—backache, arthritis, pervasive tiredness—can be put right by the right treatment. As treatments fail to restore the previous level of function and quality of life the individual becomes disillusioned with conventional medicine, and may look elsewhere, or simply give up. If this strategy becomes untenable a guarded alliance can emerge, in which the individual develops a new kind of relationship with the medical profession. The new relationship can be a positive one, in which individual doctors or nurses are seen as saviours (hero worship) or in which medical science can be championed vigorously (team playing). A middle position is one of weary resignation, in which the individual goes along with medical advice and care as the best of a bad job, without any illusions. The most guarded of guarded alliances is consumerism itself.

The producerist option

Each form of behaviour produces specific patterns of demand for and use of health services. Hero worship may generate a body of opinion that supports a given therapy or therapist, to the extent of demanding reallocation of resources towards the chosen approach and its practitioner. Team players are the life and soul of medical charities, running for hearts and lungs, parachuting for stroke victims, raising funds by any means possible. They are the backbone of support groups, the source of mentors for the newly ill, the labour force for what Julian Tudor Hart calls 'the co-production of health'. Their experience of the benefits of whatever treatment they have had, or their hope about the possibilities for better therapy in the future, makes them into ideal activists for professionally led voluntary organizations campaigning on heart disease, stroke, or diabetes. A sense of resignation may result in the withdrawal or only limited engagement of the citizen from potentially effective services, making a crisis-led intervention at a later stage a real but very disruptive possibility. This is one source of the heartsink scenarios that occur on Sunday evenings when hospitals are full, out-of-hours staff tired, and carers of difficult patients finally lose their capacity to continue and call for help, sometimes in intractable and almost impossible situations.

Traditional consumerism, derived directly from experience, has produced some of the most effective and enduring social movements around health. Medical consumers in Britain between 1979 and 1997 not only challenged professionals individually, but also collectively through the creation of pressure groups (around maternity care in particular) and the generation of new illnesses that divided medical opinion (perhaps the best example being chronic fatigue syndrome). Driven by the experiences of pain or loss, campaigning organizations began to emerge during the 1960s and 1970s to obtain redress, reshape services or challenge the assumptions underlying medical policy and practice across a broad spectrum of problems representing threats to the bodily integrity of the self or others. The successes of organizations such as the National Childbirth Trust (NCT) and the Association for Improved Maternity Services (AIMS) showed the potential for civil society to change medicine, and growth of the health-related voluntary sector took off. Two-thirds of all such consumer pressure groups in the UK appeared after 1981, especially the condition-based groups[19] such as Schizophrenia a National Emergency (SANE), Cancer BACUP, or the Stillbirth and Neonatal

Death Society (SANDS). Their founders were angry about what happened to them, perceived their problem as being poorly understood, believed that service provision was grossly inadequate and were shocked at the lack of information made available to them.[20]

The implications of this for general practice are important. First, these movements were aimed primarily at improving specialist services, and even had some support from some GPs who had spent time picking up the pieces after poorly managed encounters between patients and narrowly focused hospital clinicians. This consumerist focus on hospital practice confirmed the subaltern status of general practice to specialist medicine, but it also kept most of us out of the firing line. It also demonstrated that one aspect of industrialization—the treatment of individuals as objects—was widespread enough within hospital medicine to generate powerful responses among articulate citizens. Second, the consumer movements had significant therapeutic effects, some of which have spilled over into general practice. Cancer care is much more civilized today compared with what it was 20 years ago, and arguably childbirth more responsive to the wishes of the pregnant woman than it was when the NCT was launched. Information about long-term conditions provided by a plethora of organizations is now readily available, and can be printed during the consultations from the patient information library lodged within the electronic medical record. So it is possible that the benign effects of consumerism could change general practice directly, if the consumer movements focus on us, and if they follow the traditional path.

The new consumerism

A new form of consumerism began to appear on the political map in the first phase of the industrialization of general practice, during the 1990s. This new consumerism was not a response to adverse personal experience, but an attitude and approach that citizens could bring to bear on medical care even if they had no experience of illness, or even of medicine. These attitudes had existed before, but had been marginal, even crankish. A number of factors seemed to have made them become more prominent, and more acceptable. First, growing affluence meant that personal and corporate resources could be used in the pursuit of consumer interests, through the extension of private health insurance to 12% of the population. Sellers in search of buyers worked hard to change perceptions, thinking, and language, so that commercial medicine became 'independent', 'alternative' medicine began to be re-badged as a valid 'complementary' approach, and anti-scientific thinking legitimized. These changes in thinking were encouraged and supported by successive governments up to 1997 to stimulate change in services and in professional conduct. Public services were influenced by these pressures, with the introduction of a 'Patients' charter', the privatization of dentistry and optical services, and (of special relevance to general practice) an emphasis on developing and publicizing complaint mechanisms.

The industrialization of general practice relies on criticism of practitioners to act as a disciplinary force within medical practice. Not only would GPs have to encounter and deal with individuals disgruntled about their treatment, who felt let down by their reliance on the knowledgeable professional who had failed to solve their problem, and as a consequence had become critical of the doctor, but a whole population that approached each consultation with distrust. Many factors seem to be involved in causing this shift in consciousness, among them a growing awareness of the hazards of scientific progress, but a series of events in the late nineties and early in the twenty-first century provided an opportunity for the government to accelerate the process of harnessing consumerism to the industrialization process. They were the high profile inquiries into deaths of children undergoing cardiac surgery in Bristol,[21] the apparently widespread storage of organs from dead children, without parental consent,[22] and the ability of a single GP, Harold Shipman, to murder a large number of patients over several years without anyone noticing. All of these events were about death, and the profession's apparent indifference to (or even enthusiasm for) the deaths of patients and the utilization of their body parts for other purposes. Professional talk about patient-centred care, and accountability to the patient, appeared to be an ideological façade covering much more instrumental—even profoundly pathological—behaviour, attitudes, and relationships. Those who had harboured feelings of distrust towards medicine and the medical profession now had hard evidence that they were right to do so. Distrust generalized from the doctor whose actions or inactions could be challenged to the whole profession, which became suspect, an interest group with a hidden agenda that had no inherent right or even competence to control the medical decision-making process or police its members.

Responses to consumerism

In the 1980s and during the first phase of industrialization political ideas about consumerism in UK health services were responses to increasing demands on health services.[23] They produced changes in the way specific services were provided—we have seen this with childbirth and cancer care already, and can add mental health services to the list. The focus was on the conduct of professionals towards their patients and the quality of interactions. General practice's response to this was to emphasize the need for communications training at both undergraduate and postgraduate level, to make a more perceptive and responsive workforce, and to avoid the problem of objectification of the patient that had afflicted specialist disciplines. The wider professional response provided a variety of ways in which the patient could be engaged in making services more relevant and personalized. Consumerism has stimulated service-wide strategies of participation and community involvement[24,25] and ideas such as 'patient participation' have become commonplace in professional literature.[26] Changes in professional working at the clinical level indicate a widespread move to involve people in decisions about their own health while shifts in healthcare towards protection and promotion of health and prevention of illness further encourage self-knowledge and responsibility.[27] Nursing, midwifery, and health visiting research in particular has contributed to the evidence base for improved communication and patient decision-making in clinical care, and to the development of patient-centred services.[28] In the provision of nursing services a participation continuum has been used to relate the concepts of user involvement in decision-making to consumerist and democratic concepts of involvement.[29]

The arrival of choice

After the Bristol, Alder Hey, and Shipman inquiries the focus of government thinking shifted from quality to choice. Medical consumerism was then redefined as patients having more choice about how their care was provided and service providers being more responsive to these choices.[30] This new form of medical consumerism makes assumptions about the behaviour of help-seeking individuals that are as superficial as professional claims to have only the best interests of the patient at heart.

> As one would expect from a method rooted in the free enterprise culture of the US and the project to turn the British Welfare State into a mixed economy ... (clinical practice) ... assumes a marketplace model of interpersonal relationships—that is to say a meeting of two equal individuals coming together to agree a bargain on the exchange of goods and services. This guiding principle is interesting ... because of the detail of interpersonal thought, feeling and action that it leaves out. It proposes a vision of single persons rationally in possession of relevant information and a cool grasp of their own motivation, finding an agreeable solution to a mutually agreed definition of need.[31]

The cool grasp of motivation and needs is the missing element, because the emerging conception of the healthy self is that of a complex system in which the body is fluid and ever-changing, threatened by turbulence and instability, in a delicate relationship to its environment and other (fragile) complex systems, defended by its immune system but frighteningly vulnerable to sudden and catastrophic collapse.[16] This is the concept of the human body that best fits the experience of AIDS, and it is far removed from the mechanical system that doctors—above all, surgeons—could fix, making trust in the medical profession simply inappropriate. There are other consequences to thinking of the body as a non-linear complex system, as anthropologist Emily Martin[16] (p. 131) argues:

> The first ... might be described as the paradox of feeling responsible for everything and powerless at the same time, a kind of empowered powerlessness. Imagine a person who has learned to feel at least partially responsible for her own health, who feels that personal habits like eating and exercise are things that directly affect her health and are entirely within her control. Now imagine such a person gradually coming to believe that wider

and wider circles of her existence—her family relationships, community activities, work situation—are also directly related to her personal health. Once the process of linking a complex system to other complex systems begins, there is no reason, logically speaking, to stop.

A new model of the body

Complex systems can be resilient because their complexity can absorb damage, and allow them to repair themselves, but there can be different outcomes: 'Because control can suddenly shift from one part of the system to another and because small initial causes can have large effects, health and harmony are by no means guaranteed. Instead sudden, catastrophic eruption or collapse can, and indeed, eventually will occur'[16] (p. 132).

This risk of system collapse is reduced if the system's defence mechanism—the immune response—is sensitive and powerful. Educating and strengthening the immune response are therefore the essence of becoming and staying healthy, but there are different views on how to educate it (as there are for educating children) and (like children) immune responses are not created equal: '... if people don't have a good lifestyle or living standard, (vaccines) are very helpful ... but ... for most of the middle-class and upper-class people, [they are] total nonsense ... the "well brought up" immune system already knows most of what it needs to know ... it is a case of overkill to keep bombarding it with unneeded information'[16].

The first quotation from Emily Martin's work is uncontroversial. Every GP and practice nurse in Britain attempts to foster a sense of control in patients, encouraging healthy eating and physical activity, and promoting the sense that individuals can determine their own health, at least up to a point. The woman described in the quotation is unexceptional, because families of several generations and workplaces of different kinds do depend on the health and resilience of women as mothers, dutiful children of ailing parents, and indispensable workers.

The second quotation is congruent with medical knowledge and experience. Small changes can have profound consequences, as when a urinary tract infection that would merely hurt a 30 year old knocks an 80 year old off her feet, and complex systems do collapse, as when septicaemia precipitates multiorgan failure. The importance of this quotation lies in the way in which the idea of a cascade of events is incorporated into an everyday, lay understanding of risk.

The third quotation is familiar from consultations with parents who declined to give their children the MMR vaccine, and with patients who value alternative medicine more than allopathy. The risk of system collapse can be connected to the 'bombardment' of the immune response with 'unneeded information'. And, to make it worse, doctors cannot be relied upon to differentiate between needful and unneeded information, either because they have an uncritical relationship to the manufacturers of vaccines and medication, or because they are paid to deliver the vaccine and have to reach uptake targets to gain their income. In this view of the doctor–patient relationship, GPs are definitely knaves. In pursuit of healthier options for strengthening infant immune systems a cohort of dissenting parents reduced the overall immunity of the population, allowed preventable infectious diseases to re-establish themselves (if only briefly) in communities, and precipitated small outbreaks of measles, rubella, and mumps.

Understanding risk

At the centre of this lay thinking is a concept of risk that we need to grasp. It is tempting to attribute a bimodal concept of high or low risk to patients and a mathematical risk model to doctors, and then seek a common language in which probability can be discussed.[32] We need to be cautious about this, because citizens' understanding of risk may be more complex than ours, making us look condescending, and medical perceptions of risk may be both negative and partial, making us look out of touch with our patients' realities. Before we can talk a common language with our patients, we may need to become accustomed to the idea that risk is a social and subjective construct that is more than the probability of adverse outcome.[33] For example, the spillage of oil into the sea from a damaged tanker is experienced as a threat to those who are exposed to the oil, but also perceived as a risk to those living nearby but not exposed to direct danger. After the Sea Empress oil tanker spillage perceived risk among people living in coastal towns not exposed to the oil was associated with both increased levels of anxiety and increased reporting of symptoms unrelated to the toxic effects of oil. In towns physically exposed to oil spillage there was only increased reporting of toxicologically related symptoms. The impact of perceived risk was greater than that of physical oil exposure, involving more persons over a wider area.[34]

Similarly, the risk of fatal outcomes will be judged to be higher than it is if the causes of death are vivid and imaginable and we all tend to overestimate the risks of uncommon hazards and underestimate those of common hazards, so that a patient driving to the surgery to talk about a 'flying phobia' based on anxieties about the dangers of air travel (compared with driving) will not consider her behaviour paradoxical. Risks may be seen as highly probable but (rightly or wrongly) of low impact (e.g. measles), or highly unlikely but of high impact (e.g. autism after MMR immunization). Such risks can be seen as widespread, and be associated with modern culture's inherent vulnerabilities (e.g. through contamination of the food chain), or with violence on a mass scale, or with the sense of personal meaninglessness. How people then interpret risks will depend on their relationship to the dominant intellectual culture, with a spectrum stretching from congruence with professional authority at one end to dissenter status or fatalism at the other. Perceptions of risk may vary, and differ from the medical view, but they are not just a matter of information deficits or miscalculations of probabilities. One way we might get to grips with the new consumerism is to think in a more complex way about how patients really understand risk, and use at least three dimensions to analyse it: (1) high or low impact; (2) high or low probability; and (3) the individual's relationship to the dominant culture.

Patient and public involvement

The illnesses of modernity are multiple and changing, and medical consumerism is evolving and expanding. These changes could destabilize everyday clinical work to the extent that general practice becomes increasingly difficult for practitioners. While this is a risk, we should not overestimate it, because consumerist attitudes and behaviours are still a minority characteristic, even in the rising generations,[2] and because general practice is highly adaptable, and is already developing ways of responding to the illnesses and the consumerist challenge to professional authority. One way in which we may change is to find anticonsumerist ways of working with patients and the wider public that are consistent with our position in the (changing) public domain.

In the second phase of industrialization of general practice, since 1997, the government has worked to a broad policy agenda favouring public involvement in health and social care organization, development, and provision.[35] It was able to draw upon the experiences gained from earlier encounters with traditional consumerism, particularly about user involvement in the planning and development of healthcare,[36] in the delivery and evaluation of mental health services,[37] in change management,[38] and in guiding healthcare research.[39] The argument that patients who are well-informed about risks and uncertainties opt for treatments that are less interventionist and cheaper,[40] seems to have the ear of government. The government also seems to have valued the disciplinary effects of consumerism on professionals, using consumer feedback not only as a judgement of quality in general practice but also as a performance indicator linked to remuneration.

In doing this New Labour has accepted some assumptions that may prove to be unsound, oversimplifications of a complex issue that could compromise the changes it wants to achieve. From an ethical perspective patient autonomy is seen as a basic value and underlying premise for the provision of healthcare, and greater patient involvement is assumed to lead to better adherence to treatment recommendations and thus to better health. Patients—seen in the aggregate with an epidemiological view—are seen as rational beings who, after being informed of the relevant benefits and risks of treatment alternatives, can share in decision-making.[41] This latter viewpoint is close to a 'Wisdom of Crowds' argument, which asserts that people who can think for themselves, and are functioning more or less independently of each other and in a decentralized way, will make better decisions and judgements than experts can, provided they have a mechanism for aggregating different opinions (for example, voting).[42] We have seen how these two assumptions—involvement leads to healthier (rather than more contented) people, and that decision-making is rational from an individual as well as a social perspective—may be overoptimistic when seen from the perspective of the consultation. Not only are the health benefits of greater involvement remain unclear, but individual decision-making is not independent of media influences, peer-group suggestion, political culture and commercial pressures. Crowds may be wiser than professionals, but successive governments have avoided giving them the vote over health services. Individual patients may be wiser than professionals too, but that is not always the case.

Another example of a challengeable assumption is the 'producerist' assertion that patients are co-producers of healthcare, because their decisions and behaviour influence healthcare provision and its outcomes, but there is little evidence that such co-production improves outcomes other than satisfaction. There may be unintended consequences, including unrealistic patient expectations of what health services can deliver, defensive behaviour among professionals resulting in higher numbers of unnecessary clinical procedures, weakening of professional morale and increased costs.[43] Without completely abandoning 'producerism' as yet another example of ill-conceived ideology, we might benefit from exploring some of the possibilities and consequences of different ways of engaging with patients. A role playing exercise devised by Andrew Thompson at Edinburgh University,[44] involving submissive, dominant, and co-producer patients (the last group favouring shared decision-making) who encountered doctors with paternalist, shared decision-making and customer-as-king (information-giving) consulting styles, produced an interesting matrix of patient and doctor experiences, as shown in Table 7.1.

GPs are accustomed to changing consultation styles in response to the very different people and problems met each day in the surgery, and I suspect will not be surprised at the experiences generated in this role play. Andrew Thompson's comments on the outcomes, however, highlight their importance for an industrialized primary care service. First, few patients and no doctors liked the customer-as-king approach. Second, while shared decision-making was ideal it was also time consuming. Third, the paternalist approach was most efficient

Table 7.1 Matrix of experiences of decision-making roles for patients and doctors

Doctor's role	Patient role		
	Submissive	Shared decision-maker	Dominant (consumerist)
Paternalist	**Patient:** anger, no control, wanted more time	**Patient:** drew out views	**Patient/doctor:** forever a standoff, did not work
	Doctor: fast, efficient and uncomfortable	**Doctor:** slow, did not work	
Shared decision maker	**Patient:** involved, democratic	**Patient:** liked discussions	**Patient:** Did not feel trusted
	Doctor: difficult, depends on patient knowledge	**Doctor:** takes a lot of time	**Doctor:** Patient may regret decision and blame doctor
Customer as king information giver	**Patient:** tiring	**Patient:** Isolating	**Patient:** Nice to demand what we want
	Doctor: role not acceptable	**Doctor:** Abdication of responsibility	**Doctor:** hostage to patient

but annoyed many patients. The potential for conflict is obvious as GPs and practice nurses are encouraged by the NHS to be both patient-centred in the consultation and efficient in the delivery of care to a specified standard.

Engaging the public in primary care

What are our options in general practice when the political culture makes assumptions about the new consumerism that, at least in part, validate its core notion of choice? It seems to me that the lesson from professional responses to traditional consumerism is that we will in the long run be better off if we engage with and try to shape consumer demand. Arnstein's ladder of public involvement[45] (see Figure 7.1) has some useful pointers that could guide general practice. First, the

Rising citizen power	Citizen control	Local people plan and manage, and control funds
	Delegated power	Majority of committee places held by citizens
	Partnership	Shared decision-making
Tokenism?	Placation	Co-option, advisory role
	Consultation	Attitude and opinion surveys, etc.
	Informing	One way flow of information
Non-participation	Therapy	'Education', seek public support for plans
	Manipulation	Developed by authorities

Fig. 7.1 Arnstein's ladder applied to general practice

argument that we are accountable at an individual level to our patients is likely to categorized (using Arnstein's ladder) as 'manipulation', given the power imbalance between professionals and citizens, however informed and articulate the latter may be. Second, the promotion of patient surveys and the powerful encouragement to discuss their findings with panels of service users constitute forms of consultation that may be little more than tokenistic. Consultations that give citizens 'voice' in the management of health services 'add participation in hierarchies or networks to the other practical burdens of using healthcare, and for limited rewards'.[46] It is hardly surprising that those who come forward to exercise 'voice' in these arrangements are few in number, self-selected, and arguably unrepresentative of either health service users or the wider community. GPs are paid to go through the motions of engaging the public while the Primary Care Trust (PCT) that requires evidence of this consultative activity is firmly in the hands of government appointees. The new labour government has adopted an Old Labour attitude towards the centralization of power, and has not countenanced a Swedish-style health service managed and planned by the elected representatives of local people, perhaps because the option of making commissioners directly representative of local service users is logical but politically risky.[46]

In general practice we are not in a position to change the composition of PCTs or alter the fundamental approach of government, but we can certainly influence government policy and, as we have seen in earlier chapters, GPs are adaptable and can challenge the routines and customs of both PCTs and government across the country. While it would be a brave practice that handed control of itself to local people, or created a management board with the majority of places held by registered patients, all practices can engage in consultation exercises while simultaneously apologizing for their essentially tokenistic nature and explaining how they are trying to reduce the democratic deficit of the NHS by other means. The new superordinate stratum of GP managers can ask the PCTs for the output from their own public engagement processes and discuss the shortcoming identified with their officials, and every practice can debate the pros and cons of Public Service Trusts that could combine PCTs with local authority children's and adults' services, under local government control.

In engaging with the public at the micro-level of the practice, the meso-level of the PCT or the macro-level of government we should keep the process real, and therefore complicated by the fact that individual citizens can be consulted as real or potential consumers of specific services, citizens with an interest in local services or taxpayers with an interest in the cost and range of services. The views that individuals have may depend on the role they are put in and surveys of patient opinion are shallow if choices are disconnected from consequences. While individuals may want immediate access to the doctor of their choice (the patient perspective), their desire could change if they are asked which other individuals in their community will lose access so that they can gain it (the citizen's perspective), or what they will personally forego to obtain this level of service responsiveness (the taxpayer's perspective).

Similarly, some honesty about the purposes and potential benefits of consultation may be helpful. Is public involvement about accurate targeting of services, and the avoidance of unwanted provision (a kind of market research), or about improved take-up of services and reduction in unit costs (a kind of marketing exercise)? Is the current annual patient survey about monitoring user satisfaction, helping with the development of policies, strategies, and priorities, or a first step in closing the NHS's 'democratic deficit'? Consultation should certainly be considered when major decisions about resource allocation are going to be taken, where public views are unknown, and is often used to make a controversial decision, where there is a high level of public interest (when it may become a 'technology of legitimation'[47]). Consultations may be launched when big, expensive services exist but their value is unclear and as such is often used before denial of services to patient groups.[48] Aware of these various purposes of consultation, GPs moving into managerial roles in the industrialized system of primary care could help their general manager colleagues clarify their thoughts about the task of patient and public involvement. This shift in thinking is one of many challenges to routines and customs that could alter the framework of industrialization itself, and that is the topic of the next chapter.

References

1. Heath I. Who needs health care—the well or the sick? *BMJ* 2005; **330**: 954–6.

2. Wilkinson H, Mulgan G. *Freedom's children: work, relationships and politics for 18–34 year olds in Britain today*. London: Demos, 1995.

3. Rowe R, Calnan M. Trust relations in health care: developing a theoretical framework for the 'new' NHS. *J Health Org Manage* 2006; **20**(5): 376–96.

4. Department of Health. *Public perceptions and patient experience of the NHS: Winter 2004 Tracking Survey*. Summary report. London: Department of Health, 2004.

5. Healthcare Commission. *Variations in the experiences of patients using the NHS services in England*. London: Healthcare Commission, 2006.

6. Rao M, Clarke A, Sanderson C, Hammersley R. Patients' own assessments of quality of primary care compared with objective records based measures of technical quality of care: cross sectional study. *BMJ* 2006; **333**: 19–22.

7. Jameson F. The politics of Utopia. *New Left Rev* 2004; **January/February**: 35–54.

8. Walker A, Walker C. *Britain divided: the growth of social exclusion in the 1980s and 1990s*. London: Child Poverty Action Group, 1997.

9. Wilkinson R. Social corrosion, inequality and health. In *The new egalitarianism*. Giddens A, Diamond P (eds). Cambridge: Polity Press, 2005, pp. 183–99.

10. Benach J, Muntaner C. Precarious employment and health. *J Epidemiol Community Health* 2007; **61**: 276–7.

11. Harkonmäki K, Korkeila K, Vahtera J, Kivimäki M et al. Childhood adversity as a predictor of disability retirement. *J Epidemiol Community Health* 2007; **61**: 479–84.

12. Offer A. *The challenge of affluence: self-control and well-being in the United States and Britain since 1950*. Oxford University Press, 2006.

13. De Vogli R, Ferrie J, Chandola T, Kivimäki M, Marmot M. Unfairness, health: evidence from the Whitehall II study. *J Epidemiol Community Health* 2007; **61**: 513–18.

14. Giddens A. *Modernity and self identity: self and society in the late modern age.* Cambridge: Polity Press, 1991, pp. 169–79.

15. Hughes J, Louw S, Sabat S. Dementia: mind, meaning and the person. Oxford University Press.

16. Martin E. Flexible bodies: science and the new culture of health in the US. In *Health, medicine and society: key theories, future agendas.* Williams SJ, Gabe J, Calnan M (eds). London: Routledge, 2000, pp. 125–45.

17. Haug M, Lavin B. *Consumerism and medicine: challenging physician authority.* London: Sage, 1983.

18. Thorne SE, Robinson CA. Guarded alliances: health care relationships in chronic illness. *Image J Nurs Sch* 1989; **21**(3): 153–7.

19. Allsop J, Jones K, Baggott R. Health consumer groups in the UK: a new social movement? In *Social movements in health.* Brown P, Zavestoski S (eds). Oxford: Blackwell, 2005, pp. 57–76.

20. Allsop J *et al.* op cit p. 61.

21. Secretary of State for Health. Improving ways of giving information. The Bristol Royal Infirmary Inquiry Final Report. chapter 23, subsections 23 and 25. London 2001.

22. Department of Health. *The Report of the Royal Liverpool Children's Inquiry (the Alder Hey Inquiry).* London: Department of Health, 2001.

23. Segal L. The importance of patient empowerment in health system reform. *Health Policy* 1998; **44**: 31–44.

24. Croft S, Beresford P. 1996. The politics of participation. In *Critical social policy: a reader.* Taylor D (ed.). London: Sage, pp. 175–98.

25. Higgins R. Citizenship and user-involvement in health provision. *Senior Nurs* 1993; **13**(4): 14–16.

26. Coulter A. Paternalism or partnership? *BMJ* 1999; **319**: 719–20.

27. Kuss T, Proulx-Girouard L, Lovitt S, Katz C, Kennelly P. A public health nursing model. *Public Health Nur* 1997; **14**(2): 81–91.

28. Cody WK. Paternalism in nursing and healthcare: central issues and their relation to theory. *Nurs Sci Q* 2003; **16**(4): 288–96.

29. Hickey G, Kipping C. Exploring the concept of user involvement in mental health through a participation continuum. *J Clin Nurs* 1998; **7**: 83–8.

30. Almond P. What is consumerism and has it had an impact on health visiting provision? A literature review. *J Adv Nurs* 2001; **35**(6): 893–901.

31. Biggs S. Community care, case management and the psychodynamic perspective. *J Soc Work Pract* 1991; **5**: 71–82.

32. Misselbrook D, Armstrong D. Thinking about risk. Can doctors and patients talk the same langage? *Fam Pract* 2002; **19**: 1–2.

33. Iliffe S, Manthorpe J. Risk maps and three dimensional models: a rejoinder to Misselbrook Armstrong. *Fam Pract* 2002; **19**(6): 704–7.

34. Gallacher J, Bronstering K, Palmer S, Fone D, Lyons R. Symptomatology attributable to psychological exposure to a chemical incident: a natural experiment. *J Epidemiol Community Health* 2007; **61**: 506–12.

35. Department of Health. Health and Social Care Act. Section 11: Public Involvement and Consultation. London: Department of Health, 2001.

36. Crawford M, Rutter D, Manley C, Weaver T, Bhui K, Fulop N, Tyrer P. Systematic review of involving patients in the planning and development of health care. *BMJ* 2002; **325**: 1263–5.

37. Simpson E, House A. Involving users in the delivery and evaluation of mental health services: systematic review. *BMJ* 2002; **325**: 1265.

38. Crawford M, Rutter D, Thelwall S. *User involvement in change management: a review of the literature.* Report to NHS Service Delivery and Organisation Research and Development Programme (NHS SDO), 2003.

39. Boote J, Telford R, Cooper C. Consumer involvement in health research: a review and research agenda. *Health Policy* 2002; **61**(2): 213–36.

40. Coulter A. What do patients and the public want from primary care? *BMJ* 2005; **331**: 1199–201.

41. Grol R. Improving the quality of medical care. *JAMA* 2007; **286**(20): 2578–85.

42. Surowiecki J. *The wisdom of crowds: why the many are smarter than the few.* Little, Brown, 2004.

43. Wensing M, Elwyn G. Improving the quality of health care: methods for incorporating patients views in health care. *BMJ* 2003; **326**: 877–9.

44. Thompson A. New millennium, new values: citizen participation as the democratic ideal in health care. *Int J Qual Health Care* 1999; **11**(6): 461–4.

45. Arnstein SR. A ladder of citizen participation. *J Am Planning Assoc* 1969; **35**(4): 216–24.

46. Pickard S, Sheaff R, Dowling B. Exit, voice, governance and user-responsiveness: the case of the English primary care trusts. *Soc Sci Med* 2006; **63**: 373–83.

47. Harrison S, Mort M. Which champions, which people? Public and user involvement in health care as a technology of legitimation Social Policy and Administration. 1998; **32**: 60–70.

48. Pfeffer N, Pollock A. Public opinion and the NHS. *BMJ* 1993; **307**.

Chapter 8

What are the alternatives?

Primary care is in crisis. The behavioural and economic evidence is ubiquitous. Patients are voting with their feet and pocketbooks by going directly to emergency departments and specialists. After promoting primary care as the manager of access to specialty care, health maintenance organizations have backed off their gatekeeper strategy for such referrals ... Incomes of primary care physicians have decreased, and insurance companies are stripping payment for some types of primary care services out of benefit packages. Primary care residencies fail to attract enough applicants, while teaching hospitals continue to withdraw much-needed support for their primary care clinics. Despite primary care's proud history and theoretical advantages, the field has failed to hold its own among medical specialties.
Gordon Moore & Jonathan Showstack, Annals of Internal Medicine *(2003)[1]*

This dismal story is not confined to the USA. Only a quarter of Canadian medical graduates are choosing family medicine as a career,[2] and the Canadian healthcare system may not be functioning in its present form in another decade if the current difficulties in filling family medicine residencies continue.[3] In Sweden recruitment to general practice needs 30% of medical students to choose this career, for the discipline just to stand still, but the current trend is for only 17% to opt into primary care.[4] A debate on the future of general practice in the *Medical Journal of Australia* in 2004 began with a vignette about a fictitious, undervalued, disempowered GP, Dr Zen, working in the year 2020 in the fully industrialized world of Australian general practice. 'Regulation had reduced Dr Zen's role to pushing buttons to answer questions in an evidence based computerised diagnostic pathway. Tired, she could spend only 5 minutes with a patient. Longer consultations were punished by pay reductions. She aspired to become a taxi driver, which would provide her with the opportunity to talk to customers'[5]

In Britain, and probably in Holland and New Zealand too, general practice is less beleaguered. Our gatekeeper role still stands, our engagement in chronic disease management has increased, our public health role is expanding, our incomes have risen, recruitment to the discipline is healthy, postgraduate education is rich and flourishing. The industrialization process, for all its vicissitudes, creates many opportunities for enthusiastic doctors to innovate and experiment. We can still worry, of course, but perhaps this is a necessary counterpoint to the easy and superficial optimism of health service reformers: 'there is a real danger that we will create a flat plurality which irons out diversity: a featureless, visionless and unimaginative profession'.[6]

Uneven development

What I hope this book demonstrates is that the components of industrialization that were apparent in the incorporation of the engineering profession in the USA into industry at the beginning of the twentieth century are visible in the working experiences of British general practitioners (GPs) one hundred years later. General practice is being industrialized into primary care, but the different components are developing at different rates. Evidence-based medicine has entered the mainstream of medical thinking rapidly, perhaps because of its modification by the different interest groups that have found it useful to achieve their own objectives. Medical management remains a minority activity among GPs, although every practice is slowly being drawn into a soft bureaucracy that will shape its performance over the coming years. The specialization and skill transfers that are needed for forward integration are underway, albeit on a small scale, while mass production methods of working have been established in every practice, and seem likely to expand in their reach and impact.

All of these components are influenced and modified by professional responses. GPs are unlikely to become serfs. The risks of industrialization are evident and widely debated, perhaps more than the benefits, and the experience of the industrialization of general practice to date is full of examples of resistance to or modification of externally imposed changes. Fears that patients or professionals are being turned into things—the process of reification—are part of the pervasive anxiety of market societies,[7] and fit alongside the public preoccupation with risk. We have no need to fear that either markets or 'command and control' hierarchies will obliterate the individuality of people as patients or of GPs, because there are always ways to subvert and resist overweening power. Rudolf Klein's aphorism describing the way the NHS works remains true: 'The captain shouts his orders and the crew carries on as before'. The only qualification to this is the impact of financial incentives, which do change the way we organize ourselves and our practices, delegate work, and see patients. Gaming aside, the net benefit seems to be an improvement in the quality of clinical practice.

Chaos or coherence?

Although we may experience the changes occurring in general practice as chaotic, there is more coherence to them than appears at first sight, and there is also evidence of joined-up thinking in the National Health Service (NHS) leadership. The first phase of industrialization was a failure, but its lessons appear to have been learned, particularly about the inability of competition to preserve equity or promote efficiency, as well as the proliferation of low trust relationships.[8] NHS managers now approach general practice with a variety of governance methods, the pace of change is adapted to local settings, practitioner expertise is drawn into management, and skill transfer is promoted. Clinical governance, evidence-based medicine, forward integration and mass production work methods do fit together into a huge policy jigsaw, even if we cannot see the picture (because we are in it). The pessimistic assessment of Alan Maynard[9] that '… Governments swing from one unevaluated structure to another, ever reluctant to evaluate, learn and improve …' looks completely wrong when the reform of general practice is seen through the lens of industrialization. It is difficult to see how or why this multifaceted process would be reversed, in the absence of an alternative approach to organizing primary care that is as complex as the current thinking about clinical governance.

There are three lessons that I think we need to consider when responding to invitations to participate more enthusiastically in practice-based commissioning. The first is that GPs as a whole are adaptable and are willing to trade-off managerial control against clinical autonomy, relinquishing some of the former to retain as much as possible of the latter. What is not clear is how far these trade-off's can go, and where the limits of the non-negotiable are in clinical autonomy. Dr Zen is a caricature, but her desire to retrain as a taxi driver tells us that a line has been crossed. At the moment my computer challenges me if I prescribe ciprofloxacin, and suggest an alternative within our local 'top ten' list of antibiotics, but I can over-ride this without difficulty, discomfort, or threat. How would I respond a call from the pharmaceutical advisor as acceptable to my sense of professional competence and autonomy, on each of the (rare) occasions when I prescribe outside the local formulary?

The second lesson is that the economic organization of general practice favours local adaptability but leads to conservative decision-making about investment, and this in turn encourages government to seek market solutions when seeking to accelerate the rate of change in the health service. It also means that the practice economy has more influence on the behaviour of practitioners than professional imperatives, with the result that we behave as a group more like Le Grand's knaves than his knights, systematizing the care of long-term conditions only when financial inducements are introduced. Professionalism functions here as a catalyst or test-bed for innovation by a few adventurous or academic practitioners, who develop and test ways of systematizing care or changing clinical practice that can be later deployed for the majority within a modified general practice contract. This conservatism is a problem for us, for when our ability to contain demand decreases, as it has done so dramatically in some specialities, we do not have to hand mechanisms for correcting this, and simply seek extra resources. The escape route from this situation that preserves some elements of managerial and clinical autonomy is probably through practice-based commissioning rather than through salaried status.

The third lesson is that our place in the public domain, which has grown so secure during the second phase of industrialization that we are as a discipline closer than ever to the public sector, means that we are instinctively antimarket (except for a few real entrepreneurs). While this is an antidote to the kind of reforms that put our North American and Australian colleagues into direct competition with specialists, it is a problem for us if we persist with an unmodified dependent contractor status. Challenges from external providers and incentives that count towards a growing proportion of practice budgets—Marquand's 'market mimicry'—are likely to be effective in reshaping general practice into primary care, with our sometimes grateful acquiescence. 'To hell with the market' is therefore unlikely to rally much more than empathy, while 'to hell with the type 2 market' is too arcane to catch on as a battle cry, even though it is likely to be the principle that the majority of GPs follow in practice.

Four challenges

There are four big challenges to general practice that are emerging during industrialization.

The need to specialize, which is held back by the conservative nature of investment decision-making

To regain control of the gatekeeper function primary care needs to deploy specialist skills further forward than at present, not necessarily by performing as specialists but by employing or deploying specialist expertise in the community setting through the mechanism of practice-based commissioning. This will also be necessary if market competition increases, although the package of skills may be different. The appearance of a 'general practice with a special interest' in ENT medicine and dermatology is long overdue, and there is a need for rapid enhancement of GP skills in these domains; claims to be able to manage uncertainty are hollow when outpatient clinics are overfull with patients who could easily be managed in primary care. Imaging and possibly endoscopy need to move nearer to practices, and right into the larger ones, so that echocardiograms, ultrasound examinations and screening for gastrointestinal tract diseases can be carried out rapidly outside hospitals. Physiotherapy and podiatry on-site will improve the quality of personal care delivered to patients, with the potential for a positive feedback effect on GP knowledge and skills. Truly innovative practices will bring welfare benefits advice and social care assessment under the umbrella of general practice as well, just as they have already done with counselling.

The weakness of our arguments about having a psychosocial perspective on health and illness

The claim that GPs understand and respond to health and illness in biopsychosocial terms is repeated in recent statements[10] about the future of general practice, but the evidence for it is thin. We are much more likely to be able to describe the consequences of cytokine release than those of youthful oppositional culture on future individual well-being or of transference on the doctor–patient relationship. We are lodged firmly within a medical model and so promote exercise as therapy well beyond the evidence of its effectiveness while not employing welfare benefits advisors despite the evidence of gain that they bring to ill and vulnerable patients. The lack of our grasp of the sociology of 'high modern society' is obvious from the responses to consumerism cited in Chapter 7, despite the huge but almost entirely segregated body of knowledge within medical sociology. Psychology is more of a problem, for there is no relevant, reliable, and predictive model of individual behaviour that applies to everyday clinical work.[11] The best on offer are the Balint approach, a growing interest in 'narrative' and a handful of techniques beyond basic communications skills—modified cognitive-behavioural therapy, motivational interviewing—that some interested practitioners learn and try to employ. The Balint approach is no longer fashionable, perhaps because of its reliance on psychodynamic models of emotion and behaviour that fit uncomfortably alongside quantitative science. This may be our loss, for not only does it shed some light on interpersonal relationships but also (and unusually) talks about the pleasure of working in general practice, claiming as its essential nature:

> to add to the pleasure, satisfaction and competence of doctors in their ordinary work. The aim is not to teach a specialty ... but to leave these specialties to the specialists. The aim is to get to the heart of the matter with GPs whose burdens are great and whose satisfactions can sometimes be hidden because adequacy continues to be measured, both by GPs and patients, in terms formulated by specialists.[12]

One of the objectives of our professional body and of academic primary care might be to develop the theoretical basis and educational responses for a truly biopsychosocial model of general practice, but until that happens we should be cautious in our claims to 'holism'.

We already have the beginnings of a theoretical basis for a truly generalist perspective, in a synthesis of epidemiology, sociology of health and illness, and in (an admittedly underdeveloped) social psychology of modern societies. We can understand why some become ill while others do not, and express this as in terms of the life course, as the Figure 8.1 shows.

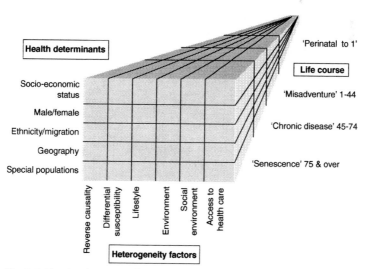

Fig. 8.1 The development of heterogeneity over a life course (modified from Hertzman et al 1994[i])

In this model health is seen as being determined by factors like socio-economic status, genetic predisposition and social environment and being modified by sources of heterogeneity, over a life course with discernable stages.[13] The factors on the vertical and horizontal axes of the matrix interact throughout life, changing the health status of the person and creating individuals who become increasingly different from each other as they get older. The older population is heterogeneous in ways that the diverse population of children is not, because more interactions have accumulated over time. This model can be used for populations and for individuals, and can be applied to the consultation as well as to the commissioning plan.

The consumerist challenge and the relative weakness of general practice in engaging with the public need to be addressed. The strategy of public engagement that the NHS is using could be the beginnings of a serious attempt to correct the health service's 'democratic deficit', and to create a bulwark of participatory democracy against the rise of individualist medical consumerism. Much of current public engagement remains tokenistic, and there is a risk that it will stay that way, making primary care vulnerable to consumerist challenges. Wise GPs will think about the ways in which they can add different methods of public engagement to their routine work, without overloading themselves and their teams with yet another difficult, time-consuming task. This is another area of weakness within general practice where

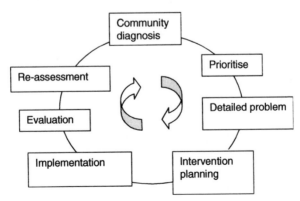

Fig. 8.2 The COPC process

much work remains to be done, perhaps through the application of community development methods[14] or COPC approaches.

The most evolved methodology for making public involvement central to service development appears to be community oriented primary care (COPC). COPC is a model of health service development which integrates public health and primary care in order to deliver targeted prioritized services to a defined population. It is an investment in the community that can reduce the 'democratic deficit' between public services and their users.[15] COPC is a method of planning, implementing, and evaluating beneficial and wanted changes in local community health and social care using a dynamic and inclusive model[16] (see the COPC cycle in Figure 8.2)

The COPC process

The tasks of each stage of the COPC cycle are:

1. **Community diagnosis.** Identifying the problem. Collect relevant demographic, economical, historical, political, and cultural data and locate human and other resources. Review the existing community/national databases, obtain the relevant demographic, social economic, mortality and morbidity data, conduct interviews, focus groups and carry out community surveys where appropriate. Unusual patterns of health or social problems in the target community should be highlighted in the analysis of the community's 'health' status. The community diagnostic process should ensure that the community's priorities are central to the next stages of the cycle.

2. **Prioritization.** A realistic, achievable number of problems to solve must be chosen by the 'community' for each turn of the cycle. This will involve debate leading to an explicit process of prioritization.

3. **Detailed problem assessment.** The short-list of problems needs to be 'worked up' in enough detail to make planning a realistic intervention possible. The academic expertise is essential to this step, both as a source of knowledge and of critical reflection.

4. **Intervention planning.** A plan for action to address the chosen problems needs to be agreed by the community.

5. **Implementation.** This entails involving the community in the implementation of the intervention and using existing

community resources wherever possible. Training of community members in skills specific to the COPC intervention will be a feature at this stage. The intervention should include short-term and long-term measurable goals.

6. **Evaluation and re-assessment.** The monitoring, evaluation, and reassessment of the COPC programme are a continuous part of the process and will generally involve a mixture of qualitative and quantitative methods to obtain the fullest possible picture of community views.

The origins of the COPC approach have parallels with the service improvement and organizational change theories proposed in the social movements literature.[17] Both involve collective action by individual volunteers with a common cause, often involving 'radical' approaches that may be in conflict with the accepted norms and 'ways of doing' things. The social movement literature proposes an alternative approach to traditional organizational change theory, incorporating the mobilization of people's own 'internal' energies, and so creating a bottom-up, locally led, 'grass-roots' movement for improvement and change.[16] Furthermore, ensuring that aims and objectives are appropriately framed can 'ignite collective action, mobilize people and inspire change'.[18]

The introduction of Primary Care Trusts has been likened to COPC,[19] partly because the community orientation develops the capacity of professionals to combine a population perspective with personal care, supports and develops teamwork processes, and extends audit to explore the needs of the local population,[20] all features of the industrialization of primary care. Furthermore, by placing the community at the centre of the development process, the issues of 'voice' and power discussed in Chapter 7 can be explicitly addressed, as they must be if communities are to be able to exert any substantial influence on primary care organizations.[21]

COPC is not a panacea for consumerism, and may be too complex for busy practitioners, or even locality commissioning groups to take on. Nevertheless it is an option for small numbers of interested practices or commissioning groups, or even Primary Care Trusts themselves, which must not underestimate the difficulties in sustaining public involvement[22] and of demonstrating its effectiveness.[23]

Exploratory work of this intensity will inevitably be done by enthusiasts in large organizations, but there are many processes for public engagement and all GPs can develop an interest in what is on the website, in the practice bulletin, or said in the patient survey.

The tendency to avoid engagement with current changes and revert to a romanticized idea about general practice

Reification—the anxiety that people are being converted into things—presumes that there was once a time when this did not happen, an invented past when Dr Findlay treated all his patients with attentive but sometimes naïve enthusiasm and Dr Cameron tempered his junior partner's modernity with a deeper and profoundly humane knowledge of human psychology.

There is a risk in British general practice that we will lapse into this kind of romanticism, perhaps by thinking that John Berger's 'A Fortunate Man' is a helpful description of a person-centred alternative to the routines of industrialized primary care. General practices can be described as being 'at the heart of their communities'[24] and GPs can be placed 'at the heart of a vibrant multidisciplinary team',[10] but these are claims to status and position that are potentially misleading and somewhat optimistic.

General practices are accessible during office hours, but at evenings and weekends NHS Direct, local out-of-hours services and Accident and Emergency departments deal with the same patients. At the moment general practice occupies the central position because it contains the only medical record that is close to being comprehensive and offers some continuity of care when other services do not, but it no longer has a monopoly role as gatekeeper to specialist services. All that is needed to reduce the centrality of general practice (short of full privatization of the health service) is the transfer of the electronic medical record from the doctor's desktop PC to the patient's smart card. Then general practices would compete with other services, American-style, perhaps trading on their main remaining asset, continuity of care. A central role in multidisciplinary teams—the beating heart, which if it stops brings down all with it—is also a slightly odd idea in the new world of industrialized primary care. Practices are grouping together or merging to manage practice-based commissioning or to see off real or imagined competitors, and the large teams containing different disciplines with variable levels of skill that are emerging from this aggregation of practitioners will be lead by GP managers, the super-ordinate stratum cultivated during the second phase of industrialization. They may well be at the heart of these teams, but the jobbing GP will not, especially if she is a salaried employee.

The future

The industrialization of general practice into primary care need not follow one path. As we have seen, the industrialization process is being made up as its protagonists go along, with ample scope for failed experiments and policy jaunts down blind alleys. At each stage a number options appear and jostle for attention, always competing with the desire to go back to the old system of organizing general practice. The only thing we can be sure about is that the NHS will continue to change. There are plenty of opinions about how this might happen, and some of them give a special role to general practice and primary care. Alison While, professor of Community Nursing at King's College London, suggests that neither staff nor users are prepared to tolerate the current situation in the NHS and points towards the solution recommended by Reform, a mixed economy of providers and enhanced primary care.[25] Another suggestion is to abandon the single payer system of the current NHS altogether and opt for competing funding bodies, so that citizens can choose to join one 'health plan' from a menu (but not choose not to join any). Competition between commissioners would focus the minds of providers, in general practice and in hospital, on cost and quality of care, and the conflict of interest in general practice commissioning (where GPs are both commissioners and providers) would be eliminated.[26]

In my view there are a number of future possibilities inherent in present trends. If maximal industrialization occurs in general practice without professional amelioration, but against a background of increasing resource constraint, we might see:

- The growth of a professionally diversified primary care work-force, with increasing part-time working, and a target-driven, impersonal work style with limited responsiveness to individuals and evident rationing of services.

- Large scale skill transfers, with nurse practitioners becoming alternatives to doctors and minimally trained staff (healthcare assistants) taking on simple nursing tasks.

- The further growth of the private medical sector, which will claim to offer the personalized service that the public sector is losing. (This claim is likely to be spurious, as the growth of the private sector is also likely to result in industrialization processes occurring within it as insurance companies seek to contain costs).

- The further growth of 'alternative medicine', which will be genuinely personal as long as it is based on individual transactions between patients and practitioners, but of limited effectiveness.

However, if general practice resists change powerfully (and is supported by other disciplines in doing so), there is likely to be:

- Less emphasis on the standardization of primary care services, and continued acceptance of some degree of variation in the quality of practice.

- A slower pace of change in general practice, and in the diffusion of knowledge and expertise.

- Professional resistance to rationalization of services and cost containment.

- Continuous conflict between professions and government over resource allocation.

- Justifications in terms of patient-centredness.

This alternative to industrialization does nothing to address the issue of resources and demand, and may be little more than a route to conflict between professionals and politicians, with failure to change the performance and character of public health services. Given the tendency to find compromise solutions at micro-, meso-, and macro-levels within the healthcare system, such conflicts may appear and be resolved piecemeal (but perhaps only partially) over a long period of time. If this occurs privatization of primary care might appear to be an acceptable alternative to continuous conflict to both government and the profession.

Leading change

It should be obvious by now that my preferred option is different to both of these, and requires the full but critical engagement of GPs in the development of clinical governance and the industrialization of general practice into primary care. The pragmatic reasons for this are that it will preserve the working autonomy of practitioners, improve the quality of medical care in the community and help ward off market solutions to the problems of the public health service. The fundamental reason is that in 'high modern society' all the processes at work in the population that were described in Chapter 7 need to be moderated by a healthcare system that does not exploit patients as a source of profit (that is, as commodities), but instead treats them as citizens of equal worth. In my view this can be achieved better by the full-on application of psychology, sociology and medical science and technology than by the elaboration of principles of patient-centredness. The onus is on the professional organizations of primary care to take leading roles in the processes of change. The Royal College of General Practitioners has a track record of innovation that will be tested by industrialization, but will need to beware of its latent romanticism, while the negotiators within the British Medical Association will need to adopt a positive attitude to change and not seek to defend forms of economic organization that limit the rate and scope of change.

Family medicine is faced with the rise of market liberalism throughout the world, giving rise to new perspectives of economic prosperity, as well as widening gaps between the rich and affluent, and a growing number of unemployed, poor, and marginalized people. Poverty and long-term unemployment are becoming permanent problems even in the rich world. The challenge to family medicine is twofold. First, to develop a broader understanding of the associations between social risk factors on a population level, and their clinical expressions in individual patients in terms of illness, sick role behaviour and manifest disease, and potential for constructive coping. Second, to maintain a system of universally available primary healthcare, meeting the needs of those who are not in the best position to pay.[27] We need not end on a pessimistic note, because general practice and family medicine still have much to offer, and could even have decisive effects on the direction of social development, but only if they can continue to evolve. As one American family physician puts it: 'In a world plagued with unforeseen discontinuities, general practice will need to maintain its core of "personal doctoring". Meeting people at the primary care level provides unique opportunities of being sensitive and responsive to unexpected changes in society, and in some areas even making contributions to the directions of change'.[27]

'Making contributions to the direction of change' is one way of describing clinical work with patients in general practice, and it requires a long-term commitment and a continuous desire to acquire new knowledge and apply it. The same applies to influencing wider change, by making social reality legible to ourselves and our communities, and by challenging the routines and habits that make up that reality.

References

1. Moore G, Showstack J. Primary care medicine in crisis: towards reconstruction and renewal *Ann Intern Med* 2003; **138**: 244–7.

2. Rachlis V. At a crossroads: the future of comprehensive care in Canada. *Can Fam Phys* 2006; **52**(11): 1375–6.

3. Dhillon P. Pride and prejudice: the future of general practice in Canada. *BC Med J* 2005; **47**(2): 89–92.

4. Eklund-Grönberg A, Stange P The future is approaching. *Scand J Primary Health Care* 2006; **24**(4): 193–5.

5. Fraser J. Professional autonomy: is it the future of general practice. *Aust Fam Phys* 2006; **35**(5); 353–5.

6. Cotton P. Fragmentation of the health service and the future of general practice. *Br J Gen Pract* 1996; 46: 555.

7. Bewes T. *Reification, or the anxiety of late capitalism*. London: Verso, 2002.

8. Thompson A. New millennium, new values: citizen participation as the democratic ideal in health care. *Int J Qual Health Care* 1999; **11**(6): 461–4.

9. Maynard A. The revolution continues. *New Econ* 1998; **5**: 207–12.

10. Royal College of General Practitioners. *The future of general practice*. A statement by the Royal College of General Practitioners. London: RCGP, 2004.

11. Bower P. Understanding patients: implicit personality theory and the general practitioner. *Br J Med Psychol* 1998; **71**: 153–63.

12. Balint E, Courtney M, Elder A, Hull S, Julian P. *The doctor, the patient and the group: Balint revisited*. London: Routledge, 1993.

13. Hertzman C, Frank J, Evans RG. Heterogeneities in health status and the determinants of population health. In *Why are some people healthy and others not? The determinants of health of populations.* Evans RG, Barer ML, Marmor TR (eds). New York: Aldine de Gruyter, 1994, pp. 67–92.

14. Murray SA, Tapson J, Turnbull L, McCallum J, Little A. Listening to local voices: adapting rapid appraisal to assess health and social needs in general practice. *BMJ* 1994; **308**: 698–700.

15. Boumbalian P, Smith D, Anderson R, Hedl J. Community Oriented Primary Care: an emerging health promotion strategy. *J Allied Health* 1991; **20**(2): 145–51.

16. Haber D. Community-oriented primary care: applying the model to a senior centre. *Fam Community Health* 1996; **18**(4): 33–9.

17. Bate P, Bevan H, Robert G. *Towards a Million Change Agents. A review of the social movements literature: Implications for large-scale change in the NHS.* London: NHS Modernisation Agency, 2004.

18. Bevan H, Edwards N. Change ideas. Dare to be different. *Health Serv J* 2004; **114**: 18–19.

19. Koperski M, Rodnick JE. Recent developments in primary care in the United Kingdom: from competition to community oriented primary care. *J Fam Pract* 1999; **48**(2): 140–5.

20. Gillam S, Miller R. COPC—a public health experiment in primary care. London: King's Fund, 1997.

21. Cawston PG, Barbour RS. Clients or citizens? Some considerations for primary care organisations. *Br J Gen Pract* 2003; **53**: 716–22.

22. Wensing M, Elwyn G. Methods for incorporating patients' views in health care. *BMJ* 2003; **326**: 877–9.

23. Brown CS, Lloyd S, Murray SA. Using consecutive Rapid Participatory Appraisal studies to assess, facilitate and evaluate and social change in community settings. *BMC Public Health* 2006; **6**: 68.

24. Lakhani M, Baker M. Good general practitioners will continue to be essential. *BMJ* 2006; **332**: 41–3.

25. While A. No choice for the NHS: reform or bust. *Br J Community Nurs* 2007; **12**(2): 90.

26. Higgins J. Health policy: a new look at NHS commissioning. *BMJ* 2007; **334**: 22–4.

27. Westin S. The market is a strange creature: family medicine meeting the challenges of the changing political and socioeconomic structure. *Fam Pract* 1995; **12**(4): 394–401.

Bibliography

Abel R. Staff implications of schemes of attachment of Local Health Authority staff (HV and Home Nursing) to General Practitioners. Study No.1 1969 DHSS Social Science Research Unit. London: HMSO.

Allen P. Clinical governance in primary care: accountability for clinical governance: developing responsibility for quality in primary care. *BMJ* 2000; **321**: 608–11.

Allsop J, Jones K, Baggott R. Health consumer groups in the UK: a new social movement? In *Social movements in health*. Brown P, Zavestoski S (eds). Oxford: Blackwell, 2005.

Almond P. What is consumerism and has it had an impact on health visiting provision? A literature review. *J Adv Nurs* 2001; **35**(6): 893–901.

Anon. *Clinical governance: from rhetoric to reality*. London: Thames Region NHSE, 1998.

Appleby J. Managers: in the ascendancy? *Health Serv J*, 1995; 32–3.

Appleton K, House A, Dowell A. A survey of job satisfaction, sources of stress and psychological symptoms amoing general practitioners in Leeds. *Br J Gen Pract* 1998; **48**: 1059–63.

Argyris C. *Overcoming organisational defences, facilitating organisational learning*. Boston, MA: Allyn & Bacon, 1990.

Arie S. Can GPs compete with big business? *BMJ* 2006; 1172.

Armstrong JS. Strategies for implementing change: an experimental approach. *Group Organ Stud* 1982; **7**(4): 457–75.

Arnstein SR. A ladder of citizen participation. *J Am Planning Assoc* 1969; **35**(4): 216–24.

Audit Commission. *Homeward bound*. London: Audit Commission, 1992.

Audit Commission. *What the doctor ordered*. London: HMSO, 1996.

Balint E, Courtney M, Elder A, Hull S, Julian P. *The doctor, the patient and the group: Balint revisited*. London: Routledge, 1993.

Banham L, Connelly J. Skill mix, doctors and nurses: substitution or diversification? *J Manag Med* 2002; **16**(4–5): 259–70.

Bate P, Bevan H, Robert G. *Towards a Million Change Agents. A review of the social movements literature: Implications for large-scale change in the NHS*. London: NHS Modernisation Agency, 2004.

Benach J, Muntaner C. Precarious employment and health. *J Epidemiol Community Health* 2007; **61**: 276–7.

Bernabei R, Landi F, Gambassi G, *et al*. Randomised trial of impact of model of integrated care and case management for older people living in the community. *BMJ* 1998; **316**: 1348–51.

Bevan G, Hood C. Have targets improved performance in the English NHS? *BMJ* 2006; **332**: 419–22.

Bevan H, Edwards N. Change ideas. Dare to be different *Health Serv J* 2004; **114**: 18–19

Bewes T. *Reification, or the anxiety of late capitalism*. London: Verso, 2002.

Biggs S. Community care, case management and the psychodynamic perspective. *J Soc Work Pract* 1991; **5**: 71–82.

Bilson A, Ross S. *Social work management and practice: systems principles*. London: Jessica Kingsley, 1999.

Bilson A, White S. Limits of governance: interrogating the tacit dimensions of clinical practice. In *Governing medicine: theory and practice*. Gray A, Harrison S (eds). Maidenhead: Open University Press, 2004.

Bodenheimer T, Wagner E, Grumbach K. Improving primary care for patients with chronic illness. *JAMA* 2002; **288**(14): 1775–9.

Bodenheimer T, Macgregor K, Stodart N. Nurses as leaders in chronic care. *BMJ* 2005; **330**: 612–13.

Boggis A, Cornford C. General practitioners with special interests: a qualitative study of the views of doctors, health managers and patients. *Health Policy* 2007; **80**: 172–8.

Boote J, Telford R, Cooper C. Consumer involvement in health research: a review and research agenda. *Health Policy* 2002; **61**(2): 213–36.

Bornstein B H, Emler AC. Rationality in medical decision making: a review of the literature on doctors' decision-making biases. *J Eval Clin Pract* 2001; **7**(2): 97–107.

Bosanquet N, Leese B. Family doctors and innovation in general practice. *BMJ* 1988; **296**: 1576–80.

Bosanquet N, Leese B. *Family doctors and economic incentives*. Aldershot: Dartmouth, 1989.

Bosma H, Peter R, Siegrist J, *et al*. Two alternative job stress models and the risk of coronary heart disease. *Am J Public Health* 1998; **88**: 68–74.

Boumbalian P, Smith D, Anderson R, Hedl J. Community Oriented Primary Care: an emerging health promotion strategy. *J Allied Health* 1991; **20**(2): 145–51.

Bower P. Understanding patients: implicit personality theory and the general practitioner. *Br J Med Psychol* 1998; **71**: 153–63.

Bowling A, Stramer K, Dickson E, Windsor J, Bond M. Evaluation of specialists' outreach clinics in general practice in England: process and acceptability to patients, specialists and general practitioners. *J Epidemiol Community Health* 1997; **51**: 52–61.

Bradley F, Field J. Letter. *Lancet* 1995; **346**: 838–9.

Bradley S, McKelvey DS. General practitioners with a special interest in public health; at last a way to deliver public health in primary care. *J Epidemiol Community Health* 2005; **59**(11): 920–3.

Bradlow J, Coulter A. Effect of fundholding and indicative prescribing schemes on general practitioners' prescribing costs. *BMJ* 1993; **307**: 1186–9.

Bristol Royal Infirmary Inquiry. Improving ways of giving information. The Bristol Royal Infirmary Inquiry Final Report. London, 2001.

Brown B, Crawford P. The clinical governance of the soul: 'deep management' and the self regulating subject in integrated community mental health teams. *Soc Sci Med* 2003; **56**: 67–81.

Brown CS, Lloyd S, Murray SA. Using consecutive Rapid Participatory Appraisal studies to assess, facilitate and evaluate and social change in community settings. *BMC Public Health* 2006; **6**: 68.

Brown, K, Williams E, Groom L. Health checks on patients 75 years and over in Nottinghamshire after the new GP contract *BMJ* 1992; **305**: 619–21.

Brownlie J, Howson A. Between the demands of truth and government: health practitioners, trust and immunisation work. *Soc Sci Med* 2005; 2006; **62**: 433–43.

Buetow SA, Roland M. Clinical governance: bridging the gap between managerial and clinical approaches to quality of care. *Qual Health Care* 1999; **8**: 184–90.

Bunn F, Byrne G, Kendall S. Telephone consultation and triage: effects on health care use and patient satisfaction *Cochrane Database Syst Rev* 2004; (4): CD004180.

Butler JR, Calnan MW. List sizes and the use of time in general practice. *BMJ* 1987; **295**: 1383–6.

Byrne D. Evidence-based: What constitutes valid evidence? In *Governing medicine: theory, practice*. Gray A, Harrison S (eds). Open University Press, 2004. pp. 81–92.

Calnan M, Butler J. The economy of time in general practice: an assessment of the influence of list size. *Soc Sci Med* 1988; **26**(4): 435–41.

Campbell S, Roland M, Wilkin D. Primary care groups: improving the quality of care through clinical governance. *BMJ* 2001; **322**: 1580–2.

Campbell S, Sheaff R, Sibbald S, Marshal M, Pickard S, Gask L, Halliwell S, Rogers A, Roland M. Implementing clinical governance in English primary care groups/trusts: reconciling quality improvement and quality assurance. *Qual Saf Health Care* 2002; **11**: 9–14.

Centre for the Advancement of Interprofessional Education Interprofessional education: a definition. *CAIPE Bull* 1997; **13**: 19.

Chant C. *Science, technology and everyday life 1870–1950*. London: Routledge, 1989.

Charlton BG. Megatrials are subordinate to medical science. *BMJ* 1995; **311**: 257.

Checkland K. Management in general practice: the challenge of the new General Medical Services contract. *Br J Gen Pract* 2004; **54**: 734–9.

Checkland P, Scholes J. *Soft systems: methodology in action*. Chichester: John Wiley & Sons, 1990.

Checkland K, Harrison S, Marshall M. Is the metaphor of 'barriers to change' useful in understanding implementation? Evidence from general medical practice. *J Health Serv Res Policy* 2007; **12**(2): 95–100.

Chevannes M. Social construction of the managerialism of needs assessment by health and social care professionals. *Health Soc Care Community* 2002; **10**(3): 168–78.

Chew CA, Wilkin D, Glendinning C. Annual assessments of patients aged 75 years and over: general practitioners' and nurses' views and experience. *Br J Gen Pract* 1994; **44**: 263–7.

Coast J, Noble S, Noble A, Horrocks S, Asim O, Peters T, Salisbury C. Economic evaluation of a general practitioners with special interests led dermatology service in primary care. *BMJ* 2005; **331**: 1444–9.

Cody WK. Paternalism in nursing and healthcare: central issues and their relation to theory. *Nurs Sci Q* 2003; **16**(4): 288–96.

Coiera E. Maximising the uptake of evidence into clinical practice: an information economics approach. *Med J Aust* 2001; **174**(9): 467–70.

Coleman P, Nicholl J. Influence of evidence-based guidance on health policy and clinical practice in England. *Qual Health Care* 2001; **10**(4): 229–37.

Corney RH, Kerrison S. Fundholding in South Thames Region. *Br J Gen Pract* 1997; **47**(422): 553–6.

Coser L. *The functions of social conflict*. New York: Free Press, 1976.

Cotton P. Fragmentation of the health service and the future of general practice. *Br J Gen Pract* 1996; **46**: 555.

Coulter A. Paternalism or partnership? *BMJ* 1999; **319**: 719–20.

Coulter A. What do patients and the public want from primary care? *BMJ* 2005; **331**: 1199–201.

Courpasson D. Managerial strategies of domination: power in soft bureaucracies. *Organ Stud* 2000; **21**(1): 141–61.

Craig N, McGregor S, Drummond N, Fischbacher M, Iliffe S. Factors affecting the shift towards a 'primary care led' NHS. *Br J Gen Pract* 2002; **52**(484): 895–900.

Crawford M, Rutter D, Manley C, Weaver T, Bhui K, Fulop N, Tyrer P. Systematic review of involving patients in the planning and development of health care. *BMJ* 2002; **325**: 1263–5.

Crawford M, Rutter D, Thelwall S. *User involvement in change management: a review of the literature*. Report to NHS Service Delivery and Organisation Research and Development Programme (NHS SDO), 2003.

Croft S, Beresford P. 1996. The politics of participation. In *Critical social policy: a reader*. Taylor D (ed.). London: Sage.

Cullum N, Spilsbury K, Richardson G. Nurse led care. *BMJ* 2005; **330**(7493): 682–3.

Davies J. How much does the scheme cost? *Fundholding* 1995; **4**(2): 22–4.

Dawson D. *Costs and prices in the internal market: markets vs the NHS Management Executive Guidelines.* Centre for Health Economics Discussion Paper No. 115. York: University of York, 1994.

De Lepeleire J, Heyrman J. Diagnosis and management of dementia in primary care at an early stage: the need for a new concept and an adapted procedure. *Theor Med Bioeth* 1999; **20**(3): 215–28.

De Lepeleire J, Heyrman J. Is everyone with a chronic disease also chronically ill? *Arch Public Health* 2003; **61**: 161–76.

De Vogli R, Ferrie J, Chandola T, Kivimäki M, Marmot M. Unfairness and health: evidence from the Whitehall II study. *J Epidemiol Community Health* 2007; **61**: 513–18.

Degeling P, Maxwell S, Iedema R. Restructuring clinical governance to maximise its development potential. In *Governing medicine: theory and practice.* Gray A, Harrison S (eds). Maidenhead: Open University Press, 2004.

Department of Health. The NHS and Community Care Act 1990. London: HMSO, 1990.

Department of Health. *Statistical Bulletin* 1994/11. HMSO.

Department of Health. *NHS modern and dependable* (Cm. 3852). London: The Stationery Office, 1998.

Department of Health. Health and Social Care Act. Section 11: Public Involvement and Consultation. London: Department of Health, 2001.

Department of Health. *The Report of the Royal Liverpool Children's Inquiry (the Alder Hey Inquiry).* London: Department of Health, 2001.

Department of Health. *Public perceptions and patient experience of the NHS: Winter 2004 Tracking Survey.* Summary report. London: Department of Health, 2004.

Department of Health. *Improving chronic disease management.* London: Department of Health, 2004.

Department of Health. *Supporting people with long term conditions: liberating the talents of nurses who care for people with long term conditions.* London: Department of Health, 2005.

Department of Health and Social Security. The Primary Health Care Team Report of the Joint Working Group of the Standing Medical Advisory Committee and the Standing Nursing and Midwifery Committee (Chairman W. Harding). London: DHSS, 1981.

Department of Health and Social Security. *Neighbourhood nursing—a focus for care.* London: HMSO, 1986.

Department of Health, Royal College of General Practitioners. *Implementing a scheme for general practitioners with special interests.* London, 2003 http://www.doh.gov.uk/pricare/gp-specialinterests/gpwsiframework.pdf/.

Dhillon P. Pride and prejudice: the future of general practice in Canada. *BC Med J* 2005; **47**(2): 89–92.

Dixon J, Lewis R, Rosen R, Finalyson B, Gray D. *Managing chronic disease: What can we learn from the US experience?* London: King's Fund Publications, 2004.

Donaldson L, Muir Gray J. Clinical governance: a quality duty for health organisations. *Qual Health Care* 1998; 7(Suppl.): S37–44.

Dowdswell G, Harrison S, Wright W. The early days of primary care groups: general practitioners perceptions. *Health, Social Care Community* 2002; **10**: 46–54.

Dowrick C. *Beyond depression.* Oxford: Oxford University Press, 2004.

Drennan V, Goodman C. Primary Care Nurses and the use of case management for people with long-term conditions. *Br J Community Nurs* 2004; 9(12): 22–6.

Drennan V, Iliffe S, Hanworth D, See Tai S, Lenihan P, Deave T. A picture of health. *Health Serv J* 2003; 113(5852): 22–4.

Drife JO. All Russian to me. *BMJ* 2006; **333**: 865.

Drummond M, Cooke J, Walley T. Economic evaluation under managed competition: evidence from the UK. *Soc Sci Med* 1997; **45**(4): 583–95.

Eddy D. Performance measurement: problems and solutions. *Health Affairs* 1998; **17**: 7–25.

Editorial. Evidence based medicine, in its place. *Lancet* 1995; **346**: 785.

Editorial. The latest official statistics. *Employing Nurses* 1996; September: 10–11.

Eklund-Grönberg A, Stange P. The future is approaching. *Scand J Primary Health Care* 2006; **24**(4): 193–5.

Elliott H, Popay J. How are the policy-makers using evidence? Models of research utilisation and local NHS policy-making. *J Epidemiol Community Health* 2000; **54**(6): 461–8.

Engel C. A functional anatomy of teamwork. In *Going interprofessional: working together for health and welfare.* Leatherard A (ed.). London: Routledge, 1994.

Engström Y, Miettinen R, Punamäki R-L. *Perspectives on activity theory.* Cambridge University Press, 1999.

Evelyn G, Hocking P, Burtonwood A, Harry K, Turner A. Learning to plan? A critical fiction about the facilitation of professional and practice development plans in primary care. *J Interprof Care* 2002; **16**(4): 349–58.

Exworthy M, Wilkinson E, McColl A, Moore M, Roderick P, Smith H, Gabbay J. The role of performance indicators in changing the autonomy of the general practice profession in the UK. *Soc Sci Med* 2003; **56**: 1493–504.

Ezzo J, Bausall B, Moerman DE, Berman B, Hadhazy V. How strong is the evidence? How clear are the conclusions? *Int J Health Tech Assess Health Care* 2001; **17** (4): 457–66.

Farrell C. Survival of the fittest technologies. *New Scientist* 1993; **137**(1859): 35–9.

Firth-Cozens J. Celebrating teamwork. *Qual Health Care* 1998; 7 (Suppl.) S3–7.

Fletcher AE, Price GM, Ng ESW, Stirling SL, Breeze E, Bulpitt CJ, Nunes M, Jones DA, Latif A, Fasey NM, Vickers MR, Tulloch AJ. Population-based multidimensional assessment of older people in UK general practice: a cluster-randomised factorial trial. *Lancet* 2004; **364**: 1667–77.

Flood RL. *Rethinking the fifth discipline.* London: Routledge, 1999.

Flynn R. 'Soft bureaucracy', governmentality and clinical governance: theoretical approaches to emergent policy. In *Governing medicine: theory and practice.* Gray A, Harrison S (eds). Maidenhead: Open University Press, 2004.

Ford S. GPs fear demise of profession's status. *Doctor* 2006; 24 October.

Foster R. *Innovation: the attacker's advantage.* Basingstoke; Macmillan, 1986.

Fowler P. Evidence based everything. *J Eval Clin Pract* 1997; **3**(3): 239–43.

Fraser J. Professional autonomy: is it the future of general practice. *Aust Fam Phys* 2006; **35**(5); 353–5.

Freeman G, Richards S. How much personal care in four group practices? *BMJ* 1990; **301**: 1028–30.

Freudenstein U. Fundholding from the inside. *Med World* 1993; **13**: 10–11.

Frusher T. Managing change: general practice and the transformation of primary care *Health Policy Rev* 2006; **3**: 44–58.

Fuat A, Hungin P, Murphy J. Barriers to accurate diagnosis and effective management of heart failure: qualitative study. *BMJ* 2003; **326**(7382): 196.

Gallacher J, Bronstering K, Palmer S, Fone D, Lyons R. Symptomatology attributable to psychological exposure to a chemical incident: a natural experiment. *J Epidemiol Community Health* 2007; **61**: 506–12.

Giddens A. *Modernity and self identity: self and society in the late modern age.* Cambridge: Polity Press, 2002.

Gilbert R, Franks G, Watkin S. The proportion of general practitioner referrals to a hospital respiratory medicine clinic suitable to be seen in a GPwSI respiratory clinic. *Prim Care Respir J* 2005; **14**(6): 314–19.

Gilbody S, Sheldon T, Wessley S. Should we screen for depression? *BMJ* 2006; **332**: 1027–30.

Gillam S, Miller R. COPC—a public health experiment in primary care. London: King's Fund, 1997.

Giuffrida A, Gosden T, Forland F, Kristiansen I, Sergison M, Leese B, Pedersen L, Sutton M. Target payments in primary care: effects on professional practice and health care outcomes. *Cochrane Database Syst Rev* 2000; (3): CD000531.

Glennester H. Competition and quality in health care: the UK experience *Int J Qual Health Care* 1998; **10**(5): 403–10.

Glennerster H, Owens P, Matsaganis M. *A foothold for fundholding.* London: King's Fund Institute, 1992.

Godsen T, Forland F, Kristiansen I, *et al.* Capitation, salary, fee-for-service and mixed systems of payment: effects on the behaviour of primary care physicians. *Cochrane Database Systematic Rev* 2000; **3**: CD002215.

Gosden T, Foreland F, Kristiansen I, Sutton M, Leese B, Giuffrida A, Sergison M, Pedersen L. Impact of payment method on behaviour of primary care physicians: a systematic review. *J Health Serv Res Policy* 2001.

Gosden T, Williams J, Petchey R, Leese B, Sibbald B. Salaried contracts in UK general practice: a study of job satisfaction and stress. *J Health Serv Res Policy* 2002.

Gosden T, Sibbald B, Williams J, Petchey R, Leese B. Paying doctors by salary: a controlled study of general practitioner behaviour in England. *Health Policy* 2003; **64**(3): 415–23.

Graham L. *On the line at Subaru-Isuzu*. Ithica, NY: Cornell University Press, 1995.

Gray A. Governing medicine: an introduction. In *Governing medicine: theory and practice*. Gray A, Harrison S (eds). Maidenhead: Open University Press, 2004.

Green S. A pivot for the practice. *Nurs Times* 1993; **89**: 42–4.

Greener I, Mannion R. Does practice based commissioning avoid the problems of fundholding? *BMJ* 2006; **333**: 1168–70.

Gregson B, *et al*. *Interprofessional collaboration in primary health care organisations*. Occasional Paper 52. London: Royal College of General Practitioners, 1991.

Grol R. Improving the quality of medical care. *JAMA* 2007; **286**(20): 2578–85.

Gross P, Greenfield S, Cretyin S, Ferguson J, Grimshaw J, Grol R, Klazinga N, Lorenz W, Meyer G, Riccobono C, Schoenbaum S, Schyve P, Shaw C. Optimal methjods for guideline implementation—conclusions from the Leeds Castle meeting. *Med Care* 2001; **39**(8): 1185–92.

Guthrie B. Continuity in UK general practice: multilevel model of patient, doctor and practice factors associated with patients seeing their usual doctor. *Fam Pract* 2002; **19**(5): 496–9.

Gutman A, Thompson D. *Democracy and disagreement*. Cambridge, MA: Harvard University Press, 1996.

Hackman J. *Groups that work (and those that don't)*. California: Jossey-Bass, 1990.

Halligan A, Donaldson L. Implementing clinical governance: turning vision into reality. *BMJ* 2001; **322**: 1413–17.

Ham C. Improving NHS performance: human behaviour and health policy. *BMJ* 1999; **319**: 1490–2.

Hardt M, Negri A. *Multitude: war and democracy in the age of Empire*. New York, Penguin, 2004.

Harkonmäki K, Korkeila K, Vahtera J, Kivimäki M *et al*. Childhood adversity as a predictor of disability retirement. *J Epidemiol Community Health* 2007; **61**: 479–84.

Harrison B. *Lean and mean*. New York: Basic Books, 1994.

Harrison S. The politics of evidence based medicine in the United Kingdom. *Policy Polit* 1998; **26**: 15–31.

Harrison S (ed.) *Evidence-based medicine: its relevance and application to primary care commissioning*. Round Table Series 59. London: Royal Society of Medicine Press, 1998.

Harrison S. *New Labour, modernisation and health care governance*. London: Political Studies Association/Social Policy Association conference on New Labour, New Health, September 1999.

Harrison S. Governing medicine: governance, science and practice. In *Governing medicine: theory and practice*. Gray A, Harrison S (eds). Maidenhead: Open University Press, 2004.

Harrison S, Mort M. Which champions, which people? Public and user involvement in health care as a technology of legitimation. Social policy and administration 1998; **32**: 60–70.

Haug M, Lavin B. *Consumerism and medicine: challenging physician authority*. London: Sage, 1983.

Hay E, Campbell A, Linney S, Wise E, and on behalf of the Musculoskeletal GPwSI Working Group. Development of a competency framework for general practitioners with a special interest in musculoskeletal/rheumatology practice. *Rheumatology* 2007; **46**: 360–2.

Healthcare Commission. *Variations in the experiences of patients using the NHS services in England*. London: Healthcare Commission, 2006.

Hearnshaw H, Harker R, Cheater F, Baker R, Grimshaw G. Are audits wasting resources by measuring the wrong things? A survey of methods used to select audit review criteria. *Qual Saf Health Care* 2003; **12**: 24–8.

Heath I. Out of hours primary care—a shambles? *BMJ* 2007; **334**: 341.

Heath I. Who needs health care—the well or the sick? *BMJ* 2005; **330**: 954–6.

Heath I, Sweeney K. Medical generalists: connecting the map and the territory. *BMJ* 2005: **331**: 1462–4.

Hertzman C, Frank J, Evans RG. Heterogeneities in health status and the determinants of population health. In *Why are some people healthy and others not? The determinants of health of populations*. Evans RG, Barer ML, Marmor TR (eds). New York: Aldine de Gruyter, 1994, pp. 67–92.

Hickey G, Kipping C. Exploring the concept of user involvement in mental health through a participation continuum. *J Clin Nurs* 1998; **7**: 83–8.

Higgins J. Health policy: a new look at NHS commissioning. *BMJ* 2007; **334**: 22–4.

Higgins R. Citizenship and user-involvement in health provision. *Senior Nurs* 1993; **13**(4): 14–16.

High impact changes for practice teams. NHS Institute for Innovation & Improvement, London 2004.

Holmes S, Gruffydd-Jones K, for the General Practice Airways group Education Sub-Committee. A proposal for the annual appraisal of, and developmental support for, General Practitioners with a specialist interest (GPwSIs) in respiratory medicine primary care. *Resp J* 2005; **14**(3): 161–5.

Honigsbaum F. *The division in British Medicine: a history of the separation of general practice from hospital care 1911–1968*. London, Kogan Page, 1979.

Hooker RS. Physician assistants and nurse practitioners: the United States experience. *Med J Aust* 2006; **185**: 4–7.

Hopayian K. The need for caution in interpreting high quality systematic reviews. *BMJ* 2001; **323**: 681–4.

Houghton K. Peak practices. *Health Serv J* 1993; **103**: 26–7.

HSC 1998/228. *The new NHS modern and dependable primary care groups: delivering the agenda.* Leeds: Department of Health, 1998.

Huntingdon J. *Social work and general medical practice.* London: George Allen and Unwin, 1981.

Huntington J, Gillam S, Rosen R. Clinical governance in primary care: organisational development for clinical governance. *BMJ* 2000; **321**: 679–82.

Hurst JW. Reforming health care in seven European nations. *Health Affairs* 1991; **10**(3): 7–21.

Hurst K. Primary and community care workforce planning and development. *J Adv Nurs* 2006; **55**(6): 757–69.

Iedema R, Jorm C, Long D, Braithwaite J, Travaglia J, Westbrook M. Turning the medical gaze upon itself: root cause analysis and the investigation of clinical error. *Soc Sci Med* 2006; **62**: 1605–15.

Iliffe S. Thinking through a salaried service for general practice. *BMJ* 1992; **304**: 1456–7.

Iliffe S. From general practice to primary care: developments in general practice 1980 to 1995 and beyond: Part 1. *Postgrad Med J* 1996; **72**: 201–6.

Iliffe S. From general practice to primary care: developments in general practice 1980 to 1995 and beyond: Part 2. *Postgrad Med J* 1996; **72**: 539–46.

Iliffe S, Manthorpe J. Risk maps and three dimensional models: a rejoinder to Misselbrook and Armstrong. *Fam Pract* 2002; **19**(6): 704–7.

Iliffe S, Munro J. New Labour And Britain's National Health Service: an overview of current reforms. *Int J Health Serv* 2000; **30**: 309–34.

Iliffe S, Gould MM, Wallace P. Assessment of older people in the community: lessons from Britain's '75 and over checks'. *Rev Clin Gerontol* 1999; **9**: 305–16.

Jameson F. The politics of Utopia. *New Left Rev* 2004; **January/February**: 35–54.

Jeffries D. Ever been HAD? *Br J Gen Pract* 2006; **56**: 392.

Jenkins S. *Accountable to none: the Tory nationalisation of Britain.* London: Hamish Hamilton, 1995.

Jenkins-Clarke S, Carr Hill R. Changes, challenges and choices for the primary health care workforce: looking to the future. *J Adv Nurs* 2001; **34**(6): 842–9.

Jennings-Clarke S, Carr-Hill R, Dixon P. Teams and seams: skill mix in primary care. *J Adv Nurs* 1998; **28**(5): 1120–6.

Jones GW, Sagar SM. No guidance is provided for situations for which evidence is lacking. *BMJ* 1995; **311**: 258.

Jones R, Bartholomew J. General practitioners with special clinical interests: a cross sectional survey. *Br J Gen Pract* 2002; **52**: 833–4.

Jones R, Rosen R, Tomlin Z, Cavanagh M-R, Oxley D. General practitioners with special interests: evolution and evaluation. *J Health Serv Res Policy* 2006; **11**(2): 106–9.

Katz D, Kahn RL. *The social psychology of organisations.* New York: Wiley, 1978.

Keaney M. Proletarianising the professionals: the populist assault on discretionary autonomy. In *The social economics of health care*. Davis J (ed.). London: Routledge, 2001.

Keeley D. Personal care or the Polyclinic? *BMJ* 1991; **302**: 1514–16.

Kenagy J, Berwick D, Shore M. Service quality in health care. *JAMA* 1999; **281**: 661–5.

Kernick D, Scott A. Economic approaches to doctor/nurse skill mix: problems, pitfalls and partial solutions. *Br J Gen Pract* 2002; **52**: 42–6.

Kharicha K, Levin E, Iliffe S, Davey B. Tearing down the Berlin Wall: social work, general practice and evidence based policy in the collaborative care of older people. *Health Soc Care Community* 2004; **12**(2): 134–41.

Kharicha K, Iliffe S, Levin E, Davey B, Fleming C. Tearing down the Berlin Wall: social workers' perspectives on joint working with general practice. *Fam Pract* 2005; **22**: 399–405.

Khunti K, Hearnshaw H, Baker R, Grimshaw G. Heart failure in primary care: qualitative study of current management and perceived obstacles to evidence-based diagnosis and management by general practitioners. *Eur J Heart Fail* 2002; **4**(6): 771–7.

Klein R. *The new politics of the NHS* (3rd edn). Longman: London 1995, p 197.

Kmietowicz Z. One year to save the NHS: what would you do? *BMJ* 2007; **334**: 181.

Knott M. Integrated nursing teams: developments in general practice. *Community Pract* 1999; **72**(2): 23–4.

Koperski M, Rodnick JE. Recent developments in primary care in the United Kingdom: from competition to community oriented primary care. *J Fam Pract* 1999; **48**(2): 140–5.

Koperski M, Rogers S, Drennan V. Nurse practitioners in general practice an inevitable progression? *Br J Gen Pract* 1997; **47**: 696–7.

Kunda G. *Engineering culture: control and commitment in a high-tech corporation*. Philadelphia, PA: Temple University Press, 1992.

Kuss T, Proulx-Girouard L, Lovitt S, Katz C, Kennelly P. A public health nursing model. *Public Health Nur* 1997; **14**(2): 81–91.

Lakhani M, Baker M. Good general practitioners will continue to be essential. *BMJ* 2006; **332**: 41–3.

Lakhani A, Coles J, Eayres D, Spence C, Rachet B. Creative use of existing clinical and health outcomes data to assess NHS performance in England: Part 1— performance indicators closely linked to clinical care. *BMJ* 2005: **330**: 1426–31.

Lam A. Tacit knowledge, organisational learning and societal institutions: an integrated framework. *Organ Stud* 2000; **21**: 487–513.

Langham S, Gillam S, Thorogood M. The carrot, the stick and the general practitioner: how have changes in financial incentives affected health promotion in general practice? *Br J Gen Pract* 1995; **45**: 665–8.

Laurent M, Reeves D, Hermens R, Braspenning J, Grol R, Sibbald B. Substitution of doctors by nurses in primary care. *Cochrane Database Syst Rev* 2005; (2): CD001271.

Lavin M, Ruebling I. Interdisciplinary health professional education: a historical review. *Adv Health Sci Educ* 2001; **6**: 25–47.

Le Grand J. Internal market rules OK. *BMJ* 1994; **309**: 1596–7.

Le Grand J. Competition, co-operation or control? Tales from the British National Health Service. *Health Affairs* 1999; **18**(3): 27–39.

Le Grand J. *Motivation, agency and public policy: of knights and knaves, pawns and queens.* Oxford University Press, 2003.

Leeder SR, Rychetnik L. Ethics and evidence-based medicine. *Med J Aust* 2001; **175**(3): 164–7.

Leese B. Impact on health authorities of the introduction of primary care groups and trusts. *Health Serv Manage Res* 2002; **15**: 40–5.

Leese B. New opportunities for nurses and other healthcare professionals? A review of the potential impact of the new GMS contract on the primary care workforce. *J Health Organ Manage* 2006; **20**(6); 525–36.

Leese B, Allgar V, Heywood P, Walker R, Darr A, Din I, West RM. A new role for nurses as primary care cancer lead clinicians in Primary Care Trusts in England. *J Nurs Manage* 2006; **14**(6): 462–71.

Lichtenstein RL. The job satisfaction and retention of physicians in organised settings: a literature review. *Med Care* 1998; **41**: 139–79.

Locock L, Regan E, Goodwin N. Managing or managed? Experiences of general practitioners in English Primary Care Groups and Trusts. *Health Serv Manage Res* 2004; **17**: 24–35.

Lucas K, Bickler G. Altogether now? Professional differences in the priorities of primary care groups. *J Public Health Med* 2000; **22**(2): 211–15.

Lynch M. Financial incentives and primary care provision in Britain: do general practitioners maximise their income? *Dev Health Econ Public Policy* 1998; **6**: 191–210.

Majeed A. Equity in the allocation of resources to general practice will be difficult to achieve. *BMJ* 1998; **316**: 43.

Mangin D, Toop L. The Quality and Outcomes Framework: what have you done to yourselves? *Br J Gen Pract* 2007: **57**: 435–7.

Marquand D. *The decline of the public.* Cambridge: Polity Press, 2005.

Marsh G, Kaim, Caudle P. *Teamwork in general practice.* London: Croom-Helm, 1976.

Marshall M, Mannion R, Nelson E, Davies H. Managing change in the culture of general practice: qualitative case studies in primary care trusts. *BMJ* 2003; **327**: 599–602.

Marshall M, Sheaff R, Rogers A, Campbell S, Halliwell S, Pickard S, Sibbald B, Roland M. A qualitative study of the cultural changes in primary care organisations needed to implement clinical governance. *Br J Gen Pract* 2000; **52**: 641–5.

Martin E. Flexible bodies: science and the new culture of health in the US. In *Health, medicine and society: key theories, future agendas*. Williams SJ, Gabe J, Calnan M (eds). London: Routledge, 2000.

Maxwell M, Heaney D, Howie JGR, Noble S. General practice fundholding: observations on prescribing patterns and costs using the defined daily dose method. *BMJ* 1993; **307**: 1190–4.

Maynard A. Competition and quality: rhetoric and reality *Int J Qual Health Care* 1998; **10**(5): 379–84.

Maynard A. The revolution continues. *New Econ* 1998; **5**: 207–12.

Mays N, Mulligan J-A, Goodwin N. The British quasi-market in health care: a balance sheet of the evidence. *J Health Serv Res Policy*, 2000; **5**: 49–58.

McCaffrey T. The pain of managing: the dynamics of the purchaser/provider split. in Foster A, Roberts Z, *Managing Mental Health in the Community*. London: Routledge 1999.

McColl A, Roderick P, Wilkinson E, Gabbay J, Smith H, Moore M, Exworthy M. Clinical governance in primary care groups: the feasibility of deriving evidence-based performance indicators. *Qual Health Care* 2000; **9**: 90–7.

McDonald R, Harrison S, Checkland K, Campbell S, Roland M. Impact of financial incentives on clinical autonomy and internal motivation in primary care: ethnographic study. *BMJ* 2007; **334**: 1357–9.

McKay J, Bowie P, Lough M. Variations in the ability of general medical practitioners to apply two methods of clinical audit: a five year study of assessment by peer review. *J Eval Clin Pract* 2006; **12**(6): 622–9.

McKee M, Sheldon T. Measuring performance in the NHS. *BMJ* 1998; **316**: 322.

Medawar C. *Medicines out of control: antidepressants and the conspiracy of goodwill*. Amsterdam: Aksant Academic Publishers 2004.

Midgley G. Systemic intervention for Public Health. *Am J Public Health* 2006; **96**(3); 466–72.

Miller C, Freeman M, Ross N. *Interprofessional practice inhealth and social care: challenging the shared learining agenda*. London: Arnold, 2001.

Misselbrook D, Armstrong D. Thinking about risk. Can doctors and patients talk the same langage? *Fam Pract* 2002; **19**: 1–2.

Moffatt MA, Sheikh A, Price D, Peel A, Williams S, Cleland J, Pinnock M. Can a GP be a generalist and a specialist? Stakeholder views of a respiratory GP with a special interest service in the UK. *BMC Health Serv Res* 2006; **6**: 62.

Moore G, Showstack J. Primary care medicine in crisis: towards reconstruction and renewal *Ann Intern Med* 2003; **138**: 244–7.

Moran P, Jenkins R, Tylee A, *et al*. The prevalence of personality disorder among UK primary care attenders. *Acta Psychiatr Scand* 2000; **102**: 52–7.

Morris R, Armstrong M. Do not overestimate the scheme's costs. *Fundholding* 1995; **4**(4): 13.

Mullen P. *Health and the internal market: implications of the white paper.* Discussion paper No. 25. Birmingham: University of Birmingham Health Services Management Centre, 1989.

Muntaner C, Benach J, Hadden W, Gimeno D, Benavides F. A glossary for the social epidemiology of work organisation: Part 1, Terms from social psychology. *J Epidemiol Community Health* 2006; **60**: 914–16.

Muntaner C, Benach J, Hadden W, Gimeno D, Benavides F. A glossary for the social epidemiology of work: part 2. Terms from the sociology of work and organisations. *J Epidemiol Community Health* 2006; **60**: 1010–12.

Murray SA, Tapson J, Turnbull L, McCallum J, Little A. Listening to local voices: adapting rapid appraisal to assess health and social needs in general practice. *BMJ* 1994; **308**: 698–700.

Mykhalovskiy E, Weir L. The problem of evidence-based medicine: directions for social science. *Soc Sci Med* 2004; **59**: 1059–69.

Neighbour R. *The inner consultation.* Newbury: Petroc Press, 1987.

Nicholls S, Cullen R, O'Neill S, Halligan A. Clinical governance: its origins and foundations. *Br J Clin Governance* 2000; **5**(3): 172–8.

Niessen L, Grijseels E, Rutten F. The evidence based approach in health policy and health care delivery. *Soc Sci Med* 2000; **51**: 859–69.

Nocon A, Leese B. The role of UK general practitioners with special clinical interests: implications for policy and service delivery. *Br J Gen Pract* 2004; **54**: 50–6.

Norman G. Evidence based medicine. *Lancet* 1995; **346**: 839.

Obholzer A. Managing social anxieties in public sector organisations. In *The unconscious at work: individual and organisational stress in the human services.* Obholzer A, Roberts VZ (eds). London: Routledge, 1994, pp. 175–6.

Ovretveit H. How to describe interprofessional working. In *Interprofessional working for health and social care.* Oevreitveit J, Mathias P, Thompson T (eds). Basingstoke: Macmillan Press, 1997.

Offer A. *The challenge of affluence: self-control and well-being in the United States and Britain since 1950.* Oxford Univeristy Press, 2006.

Ovretveit J. Essentials of multidisciplinary organisation. Uxbridge: Brunel University, 1988.

Owen P. Clinical practice and medical research: bridging the divide between the two cultures. *Br J Gen Pract* 1995; **45**: 557–60.

Paton C. Firm control. *Health Serv J* 1992; **102**: 20–2.

Payne M. *Teamwork in multiprofessional care.* Basingstoke: Palgrave, 2000.

Pearson P, Jones K. Primary care—opportunities and threats. *BMJ* 1997; **314**(7083): 817–20.

Perleth M, Jakubowski E, Busse R. What is best practice in health care? *Health Policy* 2001; **56**(3): 235–50.

Petchey R. General practitioner fundholding: weighing the evidence. *Lancet* 1995; **346**: 1139–42.

Petit-Zeman S. *Doctor, what's wrong? Making the NHS human again.* London: Routledge, 2005.

Pfeffer N, Pollock A. Public opinion and the NHS. *BMJ* 1993; **307**.

Pickard S, Sheaff R, Dowling B. Exit, voice, governance and user-responsiveness: the case of the English primary care trusts. *Soc Sci Med* 2006; **63**: 373–83.

Pinnock H, Netuveli G, Price D, Sheik A. General practitioners with a special interest in respiratory medicine: national survey of UK primary care organisations. *BMC Health Serv Res* 2005; **5**: 40.

Piore MJ, Sabel CF. *The second industrial divide: possibilities for prosperity.* New York: Basic Books, 1984.

Poulton B, West M. The determinants of effectiveness in multi-disciplinary teamwork in primary health care. *Journal of Interprofessional Care* 1999; **13**(1): 7–18.

Power M. Expertise and the construction of relevance: accountants and environmental audit. *Accounting Organ Soc* 1997; **22**(2): 123–46.

Power M. Auditing and the production of legitimacy. *Accounting Organ Soc* 2003; **28**: 379–94.

Pratt J, Gordon P, Plamping D. *Working whole systems: putting theory into practice in organisations.* London: King's Fund, 1999.

Pringle M. Clinical governance in primary care: participating in clinical governance. *BMJ* 2000; **321**: 737–40.

Pringle M, Wilson T, Grol R. Measuring 'goodness' in individuals and healthcare systems. *BMJ* 2002; **325**: 704–7.

Pritchard P. In *Inter-professional issues in community and primary health care.* Owens P, *et al.* (eds). London: Macmillan Press, 1995.

Propper C, Soderlund N. Competition in the NHS internal market: an overview of its effects on hospital prices and costs. *Health Econ* 1998; **7**(3): 187–97.

Quam L. Improving clinical effectiveness in the NHS: an alternative to the white paper. *BMJ* 1989; **299**: 448–50.

Quigley I. How much are doctors really worth: how much do doctors really earn? *BMJ* 2007; **334**: 343.

Rachlis V. At a crossroads: the future of comprehensive care in Canada. *Can Fam Phys* 2006; **52**(11): 1375–6.

Raftery J, Stevens A. Day case surgery trends in England: the influences of target setting and of general practitioner fundholding. *J Health Ser Res Policy* 1998; **3**: 149–52.

Rao M, Clarke A, Sanderson C, Hammersley R. Patients' own assessments of quality of primary care compared with objective records based measures of technical quality of care: cross sectional study. *BMJ* 2006; **333**: 19–22.

RCP, Royal College of General Practitioners and NHS Alliance. *Clinicians, services and commissioning in chronic disease management in the NHS; the need for co-ordinated management programmes.* London, 2004.

Redfern N, Stewart J. What counts is what works: postgraduate medical education and clinical governance. In *Governing medicine: theory and practice*. Gray A, Harrison S (eds). Maidenhead: Open University Press, 2004.

Rhydderch M, Elwyn G, Marshall M, Grol R. Organisational change theory and the use of indicators in general practice. *Qual Saf Health Care* 2004; **13**: 213–17.

Richardson G, Maynard A, Cullum N, Kindig D. Skill mix changes: substitution of service development? *Health Policy* 1998; **45**(2): 119–32.

Richardson J. Identifying, evaluating and implementing cost-effective skill mix. *Nurs Manage* 1999; **7**(5): 265–70.

Rigby J. Practices hit by QOF gaming accusations. *Pulse*, 2007; **7 June**.

Roberts VZ. Conflict and collaboration: managing intergroup relations. In *The unconscious at work: individual and organisational stress in the human services*. Obholzer A, Roberts VZ (eds). London: Routledge, 1994, p. 195.

Roberts VZ. The self-assigned impossible task. In *The unconscious at work: individual and organisational stress in the human services*. Obholzer A, Roberts VZ (eds). London: Routledge, 1994, pp. 112–15.

Robinson F. No private matter: taking the fight against commerce to the courts. *New Generalist* 2006; **4**(4): 58–61.

Robinson R, Le Grand J. Contracting and the purchaser-provider split. In *Implementing planned markets in health care: balancing social and economic responsibility*. Saltman RB and von Otter C (eds). Buckingham: Open University Press, 1995.

Roland M, Dusheiko M, Gravelle H, Parker S. Follow up of people aged 65 and over with a history of emergency admissions: analysis of routine admission data. *BMJ* 2005; **330**(7486): 289–92.

Roland M, McDonald R, Sibbald B, Boyd A, Fotaki M, Gravelle H, Smith L. *Outpatient services and primary care. A scoping review of research into strategies for improving outpatient effectiveness and efficiency*. Report for the NHS Service delivery, Organisation R&D Programme, London, 2006.

Rorty R. *Contingency, irony and solidarity*. Cambridge: Cambridge University Press, 1989.

Rosenberg W, Donald A. Evidence based medicine: an approach to clinical problem solving. *BMJ* 1995; **310**: 1122–6.

Rosenberg W, Donald A. Authors' reply. *BMJ* 1995; **311**: 259.

Rowe R, Calnan M. Trust relations in health care: developing a theoretical framework for the 'new' NHS. *J Health Org Manage* 2006; **20**(5): 376–96.

Royal College of General Practitioners. *The nature of general medical practice*. Report from General Practice, No. 27. London: Royal College of General Practitioners, 1996.

Royal College of General Practitioners. *The future of general practice*. A statement by the Royal College of General Practitioners. London: RCGP, 2004.

Royal College of Nursing and Royal College of General Practice. Report of the Joint Working Party on the primary health care team. London: RGCP, 1961.

Royal Pharmaceutical Society of Great Britain, BMA. *Teamworking in primary health care: realising shared aims in patient care*. London: Royal Pharmaceutical Society of Great Britain, the British Medical Association, 2000.

Ruta D, Mitton C, Bate A, Donaldson C. Programme budgeting and marginal analysis: bridging the gap between doctors and managers. *BMJ* 2005; **330**: 1501–3.

Sacket DL, Harness RBI, Tugwell P. *Clinical epidemiology: a basic science for clinical medicine*. Boston: Little & Brown, 1985.

Sacket D. Letter. *Lancet* 1995; **346**: 840.

Sackett D, Richardson W, Scott, Rosenberg, William, Haynes R. *Evidence based medicine: how to practice and teach EBM*. New York: Churchill Livingstone, 1997.

Salusbury C, Noble A, Horrocks S, Crosby Z, Harrison V, Coast J. Evaluation of a general practitioners with special interest service for dermatology: randomised controlled trial. *BMJ* 2005; **331**: 1441–4.

Scally G, Donaldson L. Clinical governance and the drive for quality improvement in the new NHS in England. *BMJ* 1998; **317**: 61–5.

Segal L. The importance of patient empowerment in health system reform. *Health Policy* 1998; **44**: 31–44.

Sennett R. *Respect: the formation of character in an age of inequality*. London: Penguin Books, 2004.

Sennett R. *The corrosion of character*. London: Norton, 1998.

Sennett R. *The culture of the New Capitalism*. Yale University Press, 2006.

Shaw B, Cheater F, Baker R, Gillies C, Hearnshaw H, Flottorp S, Robertson N. Tailored interventions to overcome identified barriers to change: effects on professional practice and health care outcomes. *Cochrane Database Syst Rev* 2005; (3): CD005470.

Sheaff R, Rogers A, Pickard S, Marshall M, Campbell S, Sibbald B, Halliwell S, Roland M. A subtle governance: 'soft' medical leadership in English Primary Care. *Sociol Health Illness* 2003; **25**(5): 408–28.

Sheaff R, Sibbald B, Campbell S, Roland M, Marshall M, Pickard S, Gask L, Rogers A, Halliwell S. Soft governance and attitudes to clinical quality in English clinical practice. *J Health Serv Res Policy* 2004; **9**(3): 132–8.

Sheard A, Kakabadse A. A process perspective on leadership and team development. *J Manage Dev* 2004; **23**: 7–106.

Shortell S, Zazzali J, Burns L, Alexander J, Gillies R, Budetti P, Waters T, Zuckerman H. Implementing evidence-based med icine—the role of market pressures, compensation incentives and culture in physician organisations. *Med Care* 2001; **39**(7): 162–78.

Sibbald B, Enzer I, Cooper C, Rout U, Sutherland V. GP job satisfaction in 1987, 1990 and 1990: lessons for the future? *Fam Pract* 2000; **17**: 364–71.

Siegrist J. Adverse effects of high-effort low reward conditions at work. *J Occup Health Psychol* 1996; **1**: 27–43.

Simpson E, House A. Involving users in the delivery and evaluation of mental health services: systematic review. *BMJ* 2002; **325**: 1265.

Smith BH. Quality cannot always be quantified. *BMJ* 1995; **311**: 258.

Smith J. *Report of the Chairman; Medical Defence Union Report, Accounts 2000.* London: MDU, 2001.

Smith J, Dixon J, Mays N, *et al.* Practice based commissioning: applying the research evidence *BMJ* 2005; **331**: 1397–9.

Smith R. Words from the source: an interview with Alain Enthoven. *BMJ* 1989; **298**: 1166–8.

Smith R, Wilton P. General practice fundholding: progress to date. *Br J Gen Pract* 1998; **48**: 1253–7.

Sorensen R, Grytten J. Contract design for primary care physicians: physical location and practice behaviour in small communities. *Health Care Manage Sci* 2000; **3**(2): 151–7.

Sorensen R, Grytten J. Service production and contract choice in primary physician services. *Health Policy* 2003; **66**: 73–93.

Southon G, Braithwaite J. *The end of professionalism.* In *Changing practice in health and social care.* Davies C, Finlay L, Bullman A (eds). London: Sage, 2000.

Spurgeon P, Hicks C, Field S, Barwell F. The new GMS contract: impact and implications for managing the changes. *Health Serv Manage Res* 2005; **18**(2): 75–85.

Sterman JD. *Business dynamics systems thinking and modelling for a complex world.* Boston, MA: McGraw Hill, 2000.

Stevenson K, Baker R, Farooqi, Sorrie R, Khunti K. Features of primary health care teams associated with successful quality improvement of diabetes care: a qualitative study. *Fam Pract* 2001; **18**: 21–6.

Stokes J. Institutional chaos and personal stress. In *The unconscious at work: individual and organisational stress in the human services.* Obholzer A, Roberts VZ (eds). London: Routledge, 1994.

Stuck AE, Beck JC, Egger M. Preventing disability in elderly people. *Lancet;* 2004; **364**: 1641–2.

Surowiecki J. *The wisdom of crowds: why the many are smarter than the few.* Little, Brown, 2004.

Tallis R. *Hippocratic oaths.* London: Atlantic Books, 2004.

Tallis R. Targets have failed the NHS. *The Times* 2006; **10 August**.

Tannenbaum S. Knowing and acting in medical practice: the epistemological politics of outcomes research. *J Health Polit Policy Law* 1994; **19**: 27–44.

Tannenbaum S. Getting there from here: evidentiary quandaries of the US outcomes movement. *J Eval Clin Pract* 1995; **1**(2): 97–103.

Tannenbaum S. Evidence and expertise: the challenge of the outcomes movement to medical professionalism. *Academic Med* 1999; **74**(12): 1259–60.

Teeling-Smith G. The economics of prescribing and under-prescribing. In *Medicines: responsible prescribing.* Wells FO (ed.). Queen's University Belfast, 1992.

Thomas P, McDonnell J, McCulloch J, While A, Bosanquet N, Ferlie E. Increasing capacity for innovation in bureaucratic primary care organisations: a whole system action research project. *Ann Fam Med* 2005; **3**(4): 312–17.

Thompson A. New millennium, new values: citizen participation as the democratic ideal in health care. *Int J Qual Health Care* 1999; **11**(6): 461–4.

Thorne M. Colonising the new world of NHS management; the shifting power of professionals. *Health Serv Manage Res* 2002; **15**: 14–26.

Thorne SE, Robinson CA. Guarded alliances: health care relationships in chronic illness. *Image J Nurs Sch* 1989; **21**(3): 153–7.

Tomlin Z, Humphrey C, Rogers S. General practitioners' perceptions of effective health care. *BMJ* 1999; **318**(7197): 1532–5.

Toner J, Miller P, Gurland J. Conceptual, theoretical and practical approaches to the development of interdisciplinary teams: a transactional model. *Educ Gerontol* 1994; **20**: 53–69.

Tudor Hart J. *A new kind of doctor*. London: Merlin 1988.

Tuohy CH. Dynamics of a changing health sphere: the United States, Britain and Canada *Health Affairs* 1999; **18**(3): 114–34.

Unger RM. *False necessity*. London: Verso, 2004.

United States Department of Labor. *What work requires of schools: a SCANS report for America 2000*. Washington DC: United States Department of Labor, 1991.

Van de Ven AH, Poole M. Explaining development and change in organisations. *Acad Manage Rev* 1995; 510–40.

van den Anker F, Bodrozic Z. Activity theory as a basis for analysing co-operative work. In *Dealing with diversity: 5th Congress of the International Society for Cultural Research and Activity Theory, Amsterdam*. van Oers, B, Wardekker W, Blom S, Elber E, Pompert B, van der Veer R (eds). 2002.

Van der Doef M, Maes S. The job demand-control (-support) model and psychological well-being: a review of 20 years of empirical research. *Work Stress* 1999; **13**: 87–114.

Wagner E. Chronic disease management: what will it take to improve care for chronic illness? *Eff Clin Pract* 1998; **1**: 2–4.

Wagner E, Davis C, Schaefer J, Von Korff M, Austin B. A survey of leading chronic disease management programs: are they consistent with the literature? *J Nurs Care Qual* 2002; **16**(2): 67–80.

Wainwright D. Disenchantment, ambivalence and the precautionary principle: the becalming of British health policy. *Int J Health Serv* 1998; **28**(3): 407–26.

Walder B, Tramer MR. Evidence-based medicine, systematic reviews in perioperative medicine—fad or necessity? *Anaethetists* 2001; **50**(9): 689–94.

Walker N, Lorimer R. Practice based commissioning: technical briefing. *Commissioning News* No. 2 February 2007. http://www.commissioningnews.com/.

Walker A, Walker C. *Britain divided: the growth of social exclusion in the 1980s and 1990s*. London: Child Poverty Action Group, 1997.

Warwicker T. Managerialism and the British GP: the GP as manager and managed. *J Manage Med* 1998; **12**(6): 331–48.

Weick KE, Quinn RE. Organisational change and development. *Annu Rev Psychol* 1999; **50**: 361–86.

Wensing M, Elwyn G. Improving the quality of health care: methods for incorporating patients views in health care. *BMJ* 2003; **326**: 877–9.

Wensing M, Elwyn G. Methods for incorporating patients' views in health care. *BMJ* 2003; **326**: 877–9.

West M, Poulton B. Primary care teams: in a league of their own. In *Promoting teamwork in primary care*. Pearson P, Spencer J (eds). London: Arnold, 1997.

West M. *Effective teamworking*. London: Sage, 1994.

Westin S. The market is a strange creature: family medicine meeting the challenges of the changing political and socioeconomic structure. *Fam Pract* 1995; **12**(4): 394–401.

Westland M, Grimshaw J, Maitland J, Campbell M, Ledingham E, McLeod E. Understanding practice management: a qualitative study in practice management *J Manage Med* 1996; **10**(5): 29–37.

Whalley D, Bojke C, Gravelle H, Sibbald B. GP job satisfaction in view of contract reform: a national survey. *Br J Gen Pract* 2006; **56**: 87–92.

While A. No choice for the NHS: reform or bust. *Br J Community Nurs* 2007; **12**(2): 90.

Wilkinson E, McColl A, Exworthy M, Roderick P, Smith H, Moore M, Gabbay J. Reactions to the use of evidence-based performance indicators in primary care: a qualitative study. *Qual Health Care* 2000; **9**: 166–74.

Wilkinson H, Mulgan G. *Freedom's children: work, relationships and politics for 18–34 year olds in Britain today*. London: Demos, 1995.

Wilkinson R. Social corrosion, inequality and health. In *The new egalitarianism*. Giddens A, Diamond P (eds). Cambridge: Polity Press, 2005, pp. 183–99.

Williams G, Flynn R, Pickard S. Paradoxes of GP fundholding: contracting for community health services in the British National Health Service. *Soc Sci Med* 1997; **45**(11): 1669–78.

Williams R. *What I came to say*. London: Hutchinson Radius, 1990.

Willis A. Who needs fundholding? *Health Serv J* 1992; **102**: 24–5.

Wright G. Evaluating the outcome of treatment: shouldn't we be asking patients if they are better? *J Clin Epidemiol* 2000; **53**(6): 549–53.

Index